Universal Coverage

CONVERSATIONS IN MEDICINE AND SOCIETY

THE CONVERSATIONS IN MEDICINE AND SOCIETY SERIES
publishes innovative, accessible, and provocative books on a range of
topics related to health, society, culture, and policy in modern America
(1900 to the present). Current and upcoming titles focus on the historical,
social, and cultural dimensions of health and sickness, public policy,
medical professionalization, and subjective experiences of illness.

SERIES EDITORS
Howard Markel and Alexandra Minna Stern,
University of Michigan

Formative Years: Children's Health in the United States, 1800–2000
edited by Alexandra Minna Stern and Howard Markel

The DNA Mystique: The Gene as Cultural Icon
by Dorothy Nelkin and M. Susan Lindee

Universal Coverage: The Elusive Quest for National Health Insurance
by Rick Mayes

*The Midnight Meal and Other Essays
About Doctors, Patients, and Medicine*
by Jerome Lowenstein

*Deadly Dust: Silicosis and the On-Going Struggle
to Protect Workers' Health*
by David Rosner and Gerald Markowitz

Universal Coverage

The Elusive Quest for
National Health Insurance

Rick Mayes

THE UNIVERSITY OF MICHIGAN PRESS

Ann Arbor

For Jennifer, Timothy and Benjamin

Copyright 2001, 2004 by Rick Mayes
New material copyright © 2004 by
The University of Michigan
Published by the University of Michigan Press 2004
First published by Lexington Books, 2001
All rights reserved
Published in the United States of America by
the University of Michigan Press
Manufactured in the United States of America
♾ Printed on acid-free paper

2008   2007   2006   2005   5   4   3   2

U.S. CIP data applied for
ISBN 0-472-11457-3 (paper)

CONTENTS

FIGURES

TABLES

PREFACE TO THE NEW EDITION

Universal coverage has become the Mount Everest of public policy in the United States—the biggest, most daunting, and often lethal challenge on the political landscape. Base camps, both public (Medicare, Medicaid, SCHIP) and private (fringe benefit of employment), have been successfully established at different points and times. But the summit remains unreached. This book's aim is to explain how and why repeated attempts at achieving universal coverage have failed. Along the way it points out the grisly remains of these attempts—the rotting political corpses and decaying legislative proposals—that litter the history of the quest for comprehensive health care reform.

Universal coverage is actually an old topic that only seems new because it cycles back on to the top of the nation's political agenda in dramatic fashion about every ten years as a "crisis." Consequently, interest among scholars and policy analysts in our nation's lack of universal coverage has existed for decades. It grew in intensity after the demise of President Bill Clinton's 1993-94 reform effort. Although this episode did not constitute the closest our country has come to having national health insurance (events in 1974 came closer), it was the most salient and optimistic environment for the issue in a generation. The resulting disappointment with the federal government and disillusionment in its ability to address this major social problem with some measure of accomplishment is still felt by many to this day. Granted, most observers doubted that Clinton's original Health Security Plan would achieve passage unscathed. But there was a widespread consensus among liberals and conservatives alike that *some* kind of substantial legislation would eventually emerge. Few anticipated what ultimately happened: total failure to pass anything.

This book places the Clinton episode in a larger historical context stretching back to the mid-1930s, when President Franklin D. Roosevelt first seriously considered including health insurance in the Social Security Act of 1935. Unlike other scholarly examinations of the topic that focus on individual political debates over national health insurance in 1934-35, 1949-50, 1964-65, 1974-75, 1979-80, or 1993-94, my intention was to include an analysis of what happened both in the intervening years and after 1994. This type of analysis provides a more comprehensive and nuanced understanding of why failure has been (and will likely remain) so persistent.

Perhaps the most valuable insight the historical approach provides is discerning the important political relationship between Social Security and national health insurance. I argue that trying to understand why the goal of universal coverage has remained so elusive without taking into account the critically influential role of Social Security is a fatally flawed approach. Social Security provided the means for achieving universal coverage after employer-provided, tax-subsidized private health insurance became the dominant mode of financing medical care in the 1950s. The program enabled social insurance advocates the only realistic way of politically overcoming the formidable array of private interests, notably the American Medical Association (AMA).

More than any other factor, Social Security made possible Medicare's seminal passage in 1965. Added to Social Security by Congress and President Lyndon Johnson, Medicare became the cornerstone upon which policymakers could incrementally reach universal coverage, while never threatening the dominant paradigm of private health insurance. On the contrary, Medicare was modeled on private health insurance—particularly Blue Cross/Blue Shield—and for that reason complemented it.

The book goes on to explain how Medicare's failure to advance program development down an incremental path ending in universal coverage was due primarily to the very factor—minimal cost control—that made for its successful passage and acceptance by the medical community in the first place. In short, the program's virtually unrestrained generosity in reimbursing doctors and hospitals led to a cost explosion that forestalled any major expansion beyond senior citizens.

Medicare also served to permanently fragment America's medical-industrial complex. This rendered ambitious, universal schemes such as Clinton's Health Security Act politically and programmatically intractable. With the advent of Medicare, a constellation of different public programs and private insurance arrangements became institutionalized. Consequently, since the early 1970s, reformers have inherited a patchwork health care system of financing and provision that politically permits only incremental change, but that requires systemic change for anything as grand as universal coverage.

My goal was to shed some light on why and how this system has come to be the daunting reality facing current and future reformers.

I received a great deal of assistance from many individuals and organizations in the writing of this book, which was originally my doctoral dissertation. I am indebted to the University of Richmond, the John Allan Love Foundation, the National Institutes of Health, the Petris Center on Healthcare Markets and Consumer Welfare at the University of California Berkeley, the Robert Wood Johnson Foundation, the Bankard Foundation, and the University of Virginia for their generous support. The direct and indirect funding they extended to me provided one of the key elements of any scholarly work—time.

My reexamination of President Clinton's failure in the book's epilogue—an earlier version of which appeared in the *Journal of Health Care Law & Policy* (vol. 7, June/July 2004)—benefited from interviews with numerous individuals who graciously shared their time and recollections with me, including: former Staff Director of the House Ways and Means Health Subcommittee, David Abernethy; President Clinton's Health Care Communications Director, Bob Boorstin; Chief of Staff to former Senate Majority Leader Bob Dole, Sheila Burke; Representative Jim Cooper; initial Senior Advisor to the Health Care Task Force, Alain Enthoven; President and CEO of the National Federation of Independent Businesses, Jack Faris; Director of President Clinton's Health Care Transition Team, Judy Feder; Senior Economist for the Clinton Health Care Task Force, Sherry Glied; former Democratic Senator from Nebraska, Bob Kerrey; former President of the Business Roundtable, John Ong; former Clinton White House Chief of Staff and Director of OMB, Leon Panetta; former Senior Medicare Analyst for the Senate Finance Committee, Lisa Potetz; former CBO Director, Robert Reischauer; former Chairman of the House Ways & Means Committee, Dan Rostenkowski; former Treasury Secretary, Robert Rubin; CMS Administrator, Tom Scully; Representative Pete Stark; former Chair of the Council of Economic Advisors, Laura D'Andrea Tyson; former HCFA Administrators, Gail Wilensky, Bruce Vladeck and Nancy-Ann DeParle; Representative Henry Waxman; and former Chairman of Prudential Insurance and Chair of the Business Roundtable's Health Subcommittee, Robert Winters. I thank the editors of the *JHCLP* for their permission to use that work in this volume.

Many individuals provided me with helpful insights and suggestions. Edward Berkowitz, one of our country's leading welfare-state historians, initially reviewed and edited the manuscript. Paul Pierson, Jacob Hacker, and Kathleen Thelen shared some of their early working papers with me, which helped structure my arguments regarding how path dependency can affect the evolution of public policy. Without knowing me, Deborah Stone graciously read this entire book and recommended that it be published. A giant in public policy studies, and health care policy in particular, Deborah has helped me tremendously.

To Martha Derthick I owe an especially large debt of gratitude. As the chair of my dissertation committee at the University of Virginia, her patience and commitment to excellence were inspiring. She continually forced me to refine the logic of my arguments by pointing out inconsistencies and weaknesses until I addressed them. Her academic reputation is legendary and well deserved. As the country's definitive Social Security scholar, she has an intimate knowledge of the subject that proved invaluable in raising the analytical level of my writing. Any errors that remain, given such first-rate mentoring, are solely my fault.

A number of colleagues and friends have contributed to my personal well-being over the years. I want to particularly express my appreciation to: Henry and Mildred Abraham, Catherine Bagwell, Farasat Bokhari, Steve Brown, Brenda and Andy Burgess, Sheila Carapico, Carol Caronna, Robert and Theodora Carey, Akiba Covitz, Ken and Terry Elzinga, Jennifer Erkulwater, Dan Gitterman, Art and Regine Gunlicks, Doug Hicks, Todd Jaussen and his family, Jimmy Kandeh, Fritz Kling, Mark Labberton, Carol Mershon, David O'Brien, John Outland, Dan Palazzolo and his family, Tracy Roof, Larry Sabato, Richard Scheffler, Herman Schwartz, Pat and Don Thiel, Rick Smith, Vincent Wang, Ellis West, John Whelan, and Stuart Yikona and his family.

Many of my students have helped me time and again by transcribing interviews, proofreading chapter drafts, and providing endless intellectual stimulation. Among others, I want to thank: Abby Emerson, Cecelia Ackerman, Jeff Vergales, Ryan Babiuch, Christian Stadler, Scott Erwin, Scott Annett, Lindsay Shore, T. R. Straub, Meredith Stewart, Sam Brumberg, Laura Liefer, Martin Hewitt, Rob Mentz, Tara Arness, Amanda Biddle, Randy De Martino, Paul Gardner, Tom Cosgrove, Brian Pagels, Virginia Page, Tracy Pintard, Christine Livingston, Kathryn Winslow, Ryan Kocher, Brian Matson, and Elise Carlin.

My interest in the economics and politics of public policy began with an inspiring individual, Mark Hearne, at Westminster Christian Academy in St. Louis. Most people can point to the first teacher in their lives who sparked an interest in a subject that charted much of their subsequent professional development. Mr. Hearne was that teacher for me. In college I was able to study and appreciate the reality of universal health coverage by being an intern for a British Member of Parliament, Jerry Hayes, who showed me the history and workings of the British National Health Service. Bobbie Kilberg provided me the opportunity to become familiar with Medicaid and other federal-state issues as my boss in the White House Office of Intergovernmental Affairs under President George Bush, Sr. My immersion into the intricacies of health care policy was provided by Fish Brown, my mentor on the American Association of Retired Persons' Health Care Team in 1994. During this time—when health care reform was at the top of the nation's public agenda—he patiently and graciously taught me the politics, economics, and history of health care policy. I try to be the excellent teacher to my students that he was to me.

I am exceedingly grateful to Ellen McCarthy at the University of Michigan Press for making this book possible. All authors should be as fortunate as I have been to work with such an excellent editor. I also wish to express my gratitude to Kelly O'Connor and Marcia La Brenz for their editorial assistance and to Howard Markel and Alex Stern as well for including my book in their series.

My mother, father, and brother have been extraordinary sources of support in every way, as have Pat and David Gilpatric. I literally cannot thank them enough for all they have done on my behalf, but I will continue trying.

My wife, Jennifer, has been invaluable to the point of being an uncredited co-author. Without her, this book would not exist. The subtle neurosis that can eat away at writers due to prolonged solitude was kept at bay because of the daily support and superb editorial services she provided. As anyone who has undertaken a major writing and research project knows, a marathon is not necessarily to the swift or to the strong, but to the steady plodders and their key supporters.

Finally, I thank God for my family, my faith, and—not least of all—my good health.

PREFACE TO THE FIRST EDITION

National health insurance is certainly not a new topic. Interest among scholars and policy elites in our nation's lack of universal coverage has existed for decades. More recently, it has grown in intensity in the years following the demise of President Bill Clinton's 1993-94 reform effort. Although this episode did not constitute the closest our country has come to having national health insurance (events in 1974 came closer), it was the most salient and optimistic environment for the issue in a generation. The resulting disappointment with the federal government and disillusionment in its ability to address this major social problem with some measure of accomplishment is still felt by many to this day. Granted, most observers doubted that Clinton's original Health Security Plan would achieve passage unscathed. But there was a widespread consensus among liberals and conservatives alike that *some* kind of substantial legislation would eventually emerge. Few anticipated what ultimately happened: total failure to pass anything.

This book places the Clinton episode in a larger historical context stretching back to the mid-1930s, when President Franklin D. Roosevelt first seriously considered including health insurance in the Social Security Act of 1935. Unlike other scholarly examinations of the topic that focus on individual political debates over national health insurance in 1934-35, 1949-50, 1964-65, 1974-75, 1979-80, and 1993-94, my intention was to include an analysis of what happened in the intervening years. This type of historical perspective provides a more comprehensive and nuanced understanding of why failure has been so persistent.

Perhaps the most valuable insight the historical approach provides is discerning the important political relationship between Social Security and national health insurance. I argue that trying to understand why the goal of universal coverage has remained so elusive without taking into account the critically influential role of Social Security is a fatally flawed approach. Social Security provided the means for achieving universal coverage after employer-provided, tax-subsidized private health insurance became the dominant mode of financing medical care in the 1950s. The program enabled social insurance advocates the only realistic way of politically overcoming the formidable array of private interests, notably the American Medical Association (AMA).

More than any other factor, Social Security made possible Medicare's seminal passage in 1965. Added to Social Security by Congress and President Lyndon Johnson, Medicare became the cornerstone upon which policymakers could incrementally reach universal coverage, while never threatening the dominant paradigm of private health insurance. On the contrary, Medicare was modeled on private health insurance—particularly Blue Cross/Blue Shield—and for that reason complemented it.

The book goes on to explain how Medicare's failure to advance program development down an incremental path ending in universal coverage was due primarily to the very factor—minimal cost control—that made for its successful passage and acceptance by the medical community in the first place. In short, the program's virtually unrestrained generosity in reimbursing doctors and hospitals led to a cost explosion that forestalled any major expansion beyond senior citizens.

Medicare also served to permanently fragment America's medical-industrial complex. This rendered ambitious, universal schemes such as President Clinton's Health Security Act politically and programmatically intractable. With the advent of Medicare, a constellation of different public programs and private insurance arrangements became institutionalized. Consequently, since the early 1970s, reformers have inherited a patchwork health care system of financing and provision that politically permits only incremental change, but that requires systemic change for anything as grand as universal coverage.

My goal was to shed some light on why and how this system has come to be the daunting reality facing current and future reformers.

I received a great deal of assistance from many individuals and organizations in the writing of this book, which was originally my doctoral dissertation. I am indebted to the John Allan Love Foundation, the National Institute of Mental Health, the Robert Wood Johnson Foundation, the Bankard Foundation, and the Department of Government and Foreign Affairs at the University of Virginia for their generous financial assistance. The funding they extended to me provided one of the key elements of any scholarly work—time.

Many individuals gave me helpful insights and suggestions. Edward D. Berkowitz, one of our country's leading welfare-state historians, reviewed and edited the manuscript for Lexington Books. John Echeverri-Gent supplied me with an abundance of constructive criticism, as well as references that proved critical in the conceptualization of the book's analytical framework. Gerard Alexander read an earlier version of the manuscript and pointed out areas where the logic needed tightening. Paul Pierson, Jacob Hacker, and Kathleen Thelen graciously shared papers of theirs with me early in the research process that significantly helped the development of my main arguments. As one of the Social Security Administration's top administrators until the mid-1970s, Arthur Hess generously shared his recollections of Medicare's implementation and early years of operation.

To Martha Derthick I owe an especially large debt of gratitude. As the chair of my dissertation committee, her patience and absolute commitment to excellence were inspiring. She continually forced me to refine the logic of my arguments by pointing out inconsistencies and weaknesses until I adequately addressed them. Her academic reputation is legendary and well deserved. As the country's definitive Social Security scholar, she has an intimate knowledge of the subject that proved invaluable in raising the analytical level of my writing. Her retirement has resulted in an irreplaceable loss to the profession. Any errors that remain, given such first-rate mentoring, are solely my fault.

Over the course of my graduate studies and postdoctoral research, a number of people have contributed to my personal well-being. I want to particularly thank Henry Abraham, Ken Elzinga, Todd Jaussen, Carol Mershon (who also read the entire dissertation as a member of my committee), David O'Brien, Jack Owen, Larry Sabato, Richard Scheffler, Herman Schwartz, and Stuart and Mwila Yikona. Thanks to them, I will always look back on my years both as a graduate student at the University of Virginia and as a lecturer and postdoctoral fellow at the University of California, Berkeley, with great fondness.

I am grateful to Jason Hallman at Lexington Books for his patience and cooperation in managing this project. As a young academic, Jason's willingness to work with me has been particularly appreciated. I am also indebted to Ginger Strader, Melissa McNitt, Kim Dennis, and Julie Olver for their assistance in bringing this book to publication.

My mother, father, and brother have been extraordinary sources of joy and support in every way, as have Pat and David Gilpatric. I literally cannot thank them enough for all they have done on my behalf, but I will continue trying.

My wife, Jennifer, has been invaluable to the point of being a virtual co-author. Without her, this book would not exist. The subtle neurosis that can eat away at scholars due to intense solitude was kept at bay because of the daily support she provided. As anyone who has undertaken a major writing and research project knows, a marathon is not necessarily to the swift or to the strong, but to the steady plodders and their key supporters.

Finally, I thank God for my family, my faith, and—not least of all—my good health.

ABBREVIATIONS

AARP	American Association of Retired Persons
AFL-CIO	American Federation of Labor–Congress of Industrial Organization
AHA	American Hospital Association
AMA	American Medical Association
CBO	Congressional Budget Office
CES	Committee on Economic Security
CPI	Consumer Price Index
DRG	Diagnosis-Related Group
GM	General Motors
HCFA	U.S. Health Care Financing Administration
HEW	U.S. Department of Health, Education, and Welfare
HMO	Health Maintenance Organization
IUD	Industrial Union Department
NCSC	National Council of Senior Citizens
NIH	National Institutes of Health
NLRB	National Labor Relations Board
OAA	Old Age Assistance
OAI	Old Age Insurance
OASI	Old Age and Survivors Insurance
OASDI	Old Age, Survivors, and Disability Insurance
OASDHI	Old Age, Survivors, Disability, and Hospital Insurance
OECD	Organization for Economic Cooperation and Development
OMB	Office of Management and Budget
PPO	Preferred Provider Organization
PPS	Prospective Payment System
SSA	Social Security Administration
SSB	Social Security Bureau
UAW	United Automobile, Aerospace, and Agricultural Workers
USA	United Steelworkers of America

CHAPTER ONE

Introduction

"Comprehensive health insurance is an idea whose time has come in America," declared President Richard Nixon in 1974. "Let us act now to assure all Americans financial access to high quality medical care."[1] President Gerald Ford repeated his predecessor's exhortation, "Why don't we write—and I ask this with the greatest spirit of cooperation—a good health bill on the statute books before Congress adjourns?"[2] Ford's successor, President Jimmy Carter, agreed, "A universal, comprehensive national health insurance program is one of the major unfinished items on America's social agenda."[3]

The contentious issue of universal health insurance coverage did not, however, originate in the 1970s. Theodore Roosevelt ran on this issue in the Bull Moose Campaign of 1912.[4] Before his death in April 1945, his cousin, President Franklin Roosevelt, called on Congress to establish an "economic bill of rights" that included a right to medical care.[5] President Harry S Truman intensified Roosevelt's demand and claimed, "In a nation as rich as ours, it is a shocking fact that tens of millions lack adequate medical care. We need—and we must have without further delay—a system of prepaid medical insurance."[6]

Most recently, President Bill Clinton renewed the quest for universal coverage, accompanied by his famous threat to Congress before a nationwide television audience in 1994: "I want to make this very clear. . . . If you send me legislation that does not guarantee every American health insurance that can never be taken away, you will force me to take this pen, veto the legislation, and we'll come right back here and start all over again."[7] According to President Clinton's press secretary at the time, George Stephanopoulos, "The president was determined . . . to succeed where FDR, Truman, Kennedy, Johnson, Nixon, and Carter had all failed, to be remembered as the president who made basic health care, like a secure retirement, the birthright of every American."[8]

1

Few issues carry so much political risk for so little political reward as health care reform. When Clinton introduced his Health Security Act to a joint session of Congress on September 22, 1993, he added his name to a long list of prominent leaders, organizations, and coalitions that have tried to achieve comprehensive reform. Frequently, these groups' efforts have been on behalf of attaining universal health insurance coverage (defined as everyone in society having at least some form of insurance against the costs of medical care).[9] When their efforts began, change often appeared imminent. However, with but one exception, the enactment of Medicare and Medicaid in 1965, they all failed. What follows is an attempt to explain why universal health insurance, arguably one of the most persistently sought after policy goals in the twentieth century, has proved so elusive in the United States.

Overview

Each country's health care system is unique. Neither the U.S. nor any other country's system is the product of one, logical policy-making experience. They are, instead, the manifestations of many years of historical development. As Ellen Immergut points out, the organizational features of public and private health insurance have been patched together by unconnected pieces of legislation, whose effects have interacted with private initiatives undertaken by a diverse group of actors. Health systems can be described with reference to layers that reflect the political and social circumstances of different historical periods.[10] As debatable as the theory of "American exceptionalism"[11] might be, the fact that the United States is the only major Western country without universal coverage lends some measure of support to the theory and attracts the continued interest of scholars and policymakers alike.

The central question of this work is: What explains the absence of universal health insurance coverage in the United States? Despite a tradition of public support for the general notion, and numerous efforts to achieve it—from consideration during the drafting of President Roosevelt's Social Security Act of 1935 to the spectacular demise of Clinton's Health Security Act in 1994—the goal remains unfulfilled. Many will find the following explanation ironic, and social insurance enthusiasts may consider it almost heretical.

In brief, there is no one politics of health care or one explanation for the lack of universal coverage; there are, instead, different patterns of politics at different stages of policy development. There has been a unique and critical relationship, however, between Social Security and the development of health insurance (both private and public). Intimidated by organized medicine in 1935, Roosevelt excluded health insurance coverage from the Social Security Act so that the program could pass in Congress. For the next three decades, the AMA continued to prevent any public, contributory health insurance scheme from passing.

By the mid-1960s, though, Social Security had evolved into the leading, if not sole, vehicle for achieving the goal of universal health insurance coverage due to its increasing political and economic influence. The program's popularity paved an alternative path for policymakers to finally overcome organized medicine's opposition to public health insurance—with the passage of Medicare in 1965. In the process, they would use Social Security to incrementally achieve the goal of universal coverage.

Policymakers' success with incremental expansion, though, also had detrimental consequences. Specifically, Social Security and Medicare's accumulated costs eventually emerged as a major impediment to the goal. Once the payroll tax was exclusively devoted to the two programs, most policymakers became convinced that they could not raise it for any additional commitments. They chose, instead, to pursue alternative financing proposals for increasing health insurance coverage, including controversial employer mandates. These necessary attempts at forging new paths of policymaking became blocked by the constellation of interests surrounding the old, institutionalized ones: the private path of tax-subsidized, employer-provided health insurance and the public path of different government programs for targeted segments of the population.

Employers, employees, and unions established the dominant private path of health insurance in the early 1950s. Over time the path became entrenched not because it was compulsory, but because the groups continually benefited by and, therefore, reinforced it.

For the public path, Medicare's passage in 1965 was a seminal achievement in social insurance. But as a contributory scheme solely for senior citizens, it also reinforced a fragmented approach of having different health insurance programs and policies for various segments of the population. The development of private health insurance for workers and their dependents and Medicare for senior citizens made subsequent attempts at major comprehensive change (e.g., national health insurance) politically unattractive and financially unfeasible. Each individual political constituency—workers, retirees, veterans, the poor— became loyal to its own health insurance program. As an example of path dependency, the development of health insurance demonstrates how preceding stages can narrow the range of possible policy outcomes and make moving off an established path, while not impossible, progressively more difficult.[12]

E. E. Schattschneider's claim that "new policies create new politics" is affirmed in the area of health care policy as in almost no other arena.[13] The relationship between Social Security and health insurance—with Social Security coming first—proved crucial. Health insurance was left in a position both secondary and, in time, dependent. Social Security's expansion paved the way for Medicare, which offered public health insurance to the retired and disabled. Yet by reinforcing the pattern of having separate public programs for individual political constituencies, it ultimately became an obstacle on the path to the last crowning step: universal coverage.[14] The irony of this argument is that the more success policymakers had with incremental expansion—made possible only by Social Security's growing popularity—the more unlikely it became that universal coverage would ever come to fruition.

As a strategy, incrementalism gave the appearance that it could eventually result in protection for everyone. But it also led to a more costly and complicated patchwork system of health care, a system less amenable to the kind of change necessary for achieving universal coverage because the costs of adapting to a different system became extremely high. "Incremental policy-making by analogy, then, linked social insurance and health insurance within the parameters of the social security model," argues Andrew Achenbaum. "This ultimately made it possible for Washington to offer health care to the elderly, but it also rendered a truly universal comprehensive plan difficult if not impossible to develop."[15]

This experience, in which policymaking promoted a configuration of elected leaders and interest groups that militated against any universal health insurance scheme, supports Margaret Weir's argument that distributional biases in particular policies "feed back" in ways that, over time, progressively block some avenues of policy, if not entirely cutting them off. Decisions at one point in time, Weir adds, can restrict future possibilities by sending policy off onto particular tracks,[16] trajectories,[17] or, as John Ikenberry calls them, "developmental pathways."[18] Health care is a revealing example. Over time, exiting off established pathways became infeasible, as Clinton's Health Security proposal demonstrated in 1993-94. In addition to the difficulties associated with the necessary politics of retrenchment, the costs of inherited programs and the numerous constituencies that developed in support of them blocked even the politics of expansion.

Why the Absence of Universal Coverage?

Many scholars of the welfare state attribute the lack of universal coverage in the United States to its being a "welfare laggard." They argue that the United States has a comparatively meager system of social welfare. This, they claim, is due to a number of general factors: a national ideology of rugged laissez-faire individualism; federalism and a weak national government (relative to European counterparts) with a high diffusion of power; the lack of a genuine labor party in national politics; historically weak levels of unionization; and the absence of a paternalistic tradition of public provision.[19] These arguments are credible and help to explain how the balance between the public and private spheres in the United States has developed. But they fail to account for certain attributes of generosity in U.S. policy. Social Security's public pension program (OASDI), compared to equivalent programs in some European countries, is more generous and universal.[20]

Most specific explanations for the absence of universal health coverage in the United States have fallen into one of three basic categories: *ideology*,[21] *interest group activity*,[22] or *institutions*.[23] Interest group activity is undeniably a key element to policy outcomes. Yet it is also helpful to move beyond the exclusive "pluralist claim that plural and balanced social pressures are the source of political decisions."[24] By incorporating the political feedback that programs and policy decisions generate, the historical approach seeks to explain why—during different periods—some interest groups were more successful than others in lobbying for the policy outcomes they wanted (or, as Immergut puts it, "translating membership strength into political results").[25]

In brief, institutions and interest groups arguably do play the most crucial policy-making roles. But if they share a common weakness as theoretical explanations, it is their static nature; they tend to exclusively address discrete policy debates in 1934-35, 1949-50, 1964-65, 1974-75, 1979-80, or 1993-94. The original contribution of this study is to include the policy feedback between the dramatic events that fostered a pattern of increasing returns, which locked in specific pathways and patterns of policymaking. The goal is to provide a more comprehensive understanding of why major policy events played out as they did. And it contributes to a growing body of research on how policies are as much an influence on political actors and processes as they are an outcome of them.[26]

Critical Junctures, Increasing Returns, and Path Dependency

As Barrington Moore, Theda Skocpol, and many others have persuasively demonstrated, history matters.[27] What comes first, observes Robert Putnam, even if it was "accidental," conditions what comes later.[28] As a result, says Richard Rose, "policymakers are usually heirs before they are choosers."[29] The historically grounded approach I employ synthesizes the tools and structure of "historical-institutionalism"[30] and "analytical narratives,"[31] in which time provides the key dimension of comparison. Time is enormously consequential, as Dietrich Rueschemeyer, Evelyne Stephens and John Stephens have demonstrated, because "causal analysis is inherently sequence analysis."[32]

Accordingly, my approach emphasizes the influence of critical junctures, the increasing returns that follow them, and the path dependency these returns can engender. This style of analysis provides a more nuanced explanation, Daniel J. Goldhagen notes, by breaking down complex phenomena into their component parts, not only for the sake of clarity, but also for elucidating various aspects of incremental change, its ebbs and flows, and the consequences of critical junctures.[33] In understanding why policymakers pursue a particular strategy (and why they fail or succeed), the decisions of previous actors and the reasons they made them are crucial.

Critical junctures may be defined as periods of significant change that produce distinct legacies.[34] "Big historical events have big historical consequences," notes Jacob Hacker, "as these crucial periods of transition shape processes of political and economic development for decades to come."[35]

Increasing returns ordinarily follow critical junctures. They are the normal self-reinforcing effects inherent in any policy that achieves passage and is implemented.[36] Each step along a particular path strengthens these increasing returns, which makes the path more attractive for the next round. As Paul Pierson claims, "If such effects begin to accumulate, they generate a powerful (or vicious) cycle of self-reinforcing activity."[37] The basic logic of increasing returns processes can be captured in a simple mathematical illustration.[38] Imagine a standard BINGO raffle basket containing two marbles: one blue, one yellow. Blindfold an individual, spin the basket, and then have the individual reach in and randomly remove one of the marbles. Afterward, replace the original marble and add another marble of the same color. Repeat this process until the basket fills up with hundreds or thousands of marbles. Regardless of what the eventual distribution becomes in any given trial, the initial selections are critical. After the first ten, twenty, or thirty selections, the eventual equilibrium of yellow and blue marbles becomes virtually fixed, with later selections in the process altering the equilibrium only minutely, if at all.[39]

On a more anecdotal level, increasing returns help to explain why most seniors in college who happen to not like their chosen majors refuse to change them prior to graduating, even though they still have the opportunity to do so. The financial costs and additional time needed to change ("exit") from their current majors to different ones are considerable by the time they are seniors. So they usually continue along the academic paths most of them chose as sophomores. Staying in the academy, the effect of increasing returns constitutes an explanation for why numerous senior professors continue to use typewriters and calculators for the bulk of their writing and grade computing, respectively (along with graduate students if they can manage it), even though they could very well use much quicker word processors and spreadsheets. For many of them, the short-term time requirements or personal costs required to learn a new technology, such as computers, outweigh the potential long-term gains in efficiency.

As applied to the political arena of social policy, Pierson explains, there are three features intrinsically associated with increasing returns:

1) *Large set-up or fixed costs.* These create a high payoff for further investments in a given program or policy. When set-up or fixed costs are high, individuals and organizations have a strong incentive to identify and stick with a single option.

2) *Learning effects.* Knowledge gained in the operation of complex programs and policy arrangements (public and private) also leads to higher returns from continuing them. With repetition, individuals and organizations learn how to maximize the return on their investments in these complex programs and policy arrangements and are likely to spur further innovations in them.

3) *Coordination and adaptive effects.* These occur when the benefits an individual or organization receives from a particular program or policy arrangement increase as others adopt the same choices. This enhanced appeal attracts more users, reinforcing the existing advantage. Individuals and organizations will feel a need to pick the most beneficial program or policy arrangement available, because alternatives that fail to win broad acceptance will have drawbacks later on. So projections about future costs and benefits will lead individuals and organizations to adapt their actions in ways that help to make the paths that are already attractive and advantageous even more so.[40]

The more pronounced increasing return features become, the more likely it is that a particular policy area will become path dependent. Why? Because the benefits of sticking with a specific program or policy arrangement increase, as do the costs of dramatically departing or exiting from them. With the relatively short time horizons involved in public and private decision making, actors will tend to follow the path already established and adjust their behavior at the margins rather than the other way around.[41]

Roughly analogous to Charles Darwin's theory of natural selection,[42] society's institutional landscape progressively changes through the preservation of those policies and programs best adapted to survive the political competition for existence. Policies and programs that political actors choose at all tend to survive, and some thrive because of the immense amount of "sunk costs" surrounding them that make change increasingly unattractive.[43] In effect, path dependency is the end product of policymakers having "strong incentives to focus on a single alternative, and to continue moving down a specific path once initial steps are taken in that direction."[44]

It must be noted, however, that not all policy areas bear significant evidence of path dependency. Policy areas become more or less path dependent and some not at all. The condition depends upon a complex combination of factors, including, among others, whether the programs in a given policy area are entitlements or need-based welfare, whether beneficiaries involved are concentrated or diffuse, and how long the policy's time horizon is. Furthermore, determining whether a policy area becomes path dependent is done by means of inductive, not deductive, analysis. In other words, it is only after exhaustively reviewing the historical evolution of a policy that one sees either more or less evidence for path dependency; it is not assumed a priori. Thus, path dependency in any policy area is a condition that can easily evolve if given sufficient time, but does not necessarily do so universally.

Organization

The structure of this work is designed to delineate the different stages of health care policymaking, during which universal coverage became increasingly elusive. The first several chapters cover the initial stage of failure and frustration from the mid-1930s to the early 1960s. Chapter 2 focuses on the passage of Social Security—unquestionably the American welfare state's most critical juncture—and the two development pathways it initiated. The first path, old age pensions, became primarily public and produced the eventual ascendancy of old age and survivors insurance (OASI). Policymakers subordinated health insurance to old age insurance for political reasons, thereby relegating it almost entirely to the private sector.

Critical junctures of Social Security's magnitude are exceedingly rare in history, so their significance is difficult to overestimate. Because the welfare state at this time was in its infancy or formative period, interest group activity was the leading type of policy feedback[45] (with the AMA dominating). The two other leading forms of policy feedback, lock-in effects and policy learning, were virtually nonexistent, because nothing was locked in yet, nor was there much opportunity for either positive or negative experiential learning (table 1.1). Policymakers focused their political capital and energy on trying to implement and secure their legislative achievements.

Chapter 3 examines how the succeeding period—the late 1930s to 1950—reaffirmed the original decision in 1935. During this time the two policy areas continued to diverge in keeping with the initial decision: the one, OASI, becoming more solidly public, the other, health insurance, being repeatedly rejected as a public program. By 1950, policymakers had secured the public path for old age insurance, which then had comprehensive coverage and was secure against its welfare-based rival, OAA. At the same time, public health insurance had been decisively rejected due primarily to organized medicine's effective lobbying. Policymakers subsequently shifted their attention to the possibility of a private path for protecting individuals from the costs of medical care.

Roughly akin to a second critical juncture, organized labor turned to collective bargaining in 1949-50, which became the foundation for health insurance's private pathway. The NLRB facilitated this development in 1948, when it ruled that employers could offer health insurance as a fringe benefit to their employees. The NLRB's ruling effectively exempted employer-sponsored health insurance from federal taxation.[46] With collective bargaining—and the related tax advantage of health insurance defined as a fringe benefit—unions and employers made the private path a positive choice and an institution was created.

Chapter 4 describes the phase of increasing returns associated with both paths from the early 1950s to the early 1960s. The public path, Social Security, became the beneficiary of political actors' successful program building, which greatly enlarged the scheme's scope and generosity. Benefit increases were now enacted routinely. When the Eisenhower administration arrived, critics of Social Security considered the possibility of "exiting" to a new path, but quickly ruled it out as infeasible. By this time, the effects of the 1939 and 1950 amendments made any exit from the program's public path politically unattractive, if not an impossibility. So effective were Social Security's increasing returns (both political and financial) that, even during a Republican administration, disability insurance was enacted in 1956.

Meanwhile, the private path of health insurance became institutionalized mostly through collective bargaining between employers and unions. Blue Cross/Blue Shield and for-profit insurance skyrocketed, but did not attain universality. Employer-financed health insurance left out those people who did not have big and/or unionized employers: the retired, the self-employed, employees of small businesses, and the unemployed. In combination with the vigorous development of OASI (OASDI after the passage of disability insurance in 1956), this shortcoming created the possibility of opening a public path of health insurance as a complement to the established public program and as a remedy for a defect in the private sector.

Chapter 5 explains the partial success policymakers had from the mid-1960s to the early 1970s in attaching a public health insurance program to Social Security. As a product of policy learning, incremental expansion and its gradualist tactics emerged triumphant (table 1.1).[47] Lyndon Johnson's massive electoral victory in 1964 opened a window of opportunity[48] for public health insurance advocates, which they took advantage of by piggybacking Medicare onto Social Security, the welfare state's main vehicle. Further steps by policymakers along this path of incrementalism culminated in the extension of Medicare coverage to recipients of disability insurance in 1972.

As Martha Derthick has documented, this is the story of political actors successfully attaching health insurance as an increment to a well-established and then still very popular program, OASDI. The thirty previous years of failure and frustration for health insurance were years of extremely successful program building for Social Security. Health insurance became an heir to that success.[49] At the same time, path dependency can be seen in how policymakers were forced to coordinate or adapt Medicare's design to existing arrangements in the private sector. As evidence of the path's strong inertia, Medicare's (and to a lesser extent Medicaid's) payment structure largely extended the private system's third-party reimbursement model to senior citizens (and the poor) via public programs. Medicare, in particular, emerged as virtually a public Blue Cross/Blue Shield program for senior citizens, many of whom had been enrolled in Blue Cross/Blue Shield schemes during their years of employment.

Chapters 6 and 7 address the return of failure and frustration for health care reformers from the mid-1970s to the present. Chapter 6 examines how efforts to expand Medicare's coverage, which had been many proponents' unspoken goal since the program's formation,[50] became eclipsed by the program's rapidly escalating costs. Alternative means for universal coverage—notably propounded in President Nixon's employer mandate plan—failed due to organized labor's refusal to compromise its advocacy of pure social insurance expansion. Further incremental expansion along the path established by Medicare became subordinated to the more urgent goal of cost containment. Finally, the administrative relationship between Medicare and its parent program, Social Security, grew so problematic that Medicare ceased to be an add-on and became a separate program in its own right and with its own administrator, the Health Care Financing Administration (HCFA).

Addressed in chapter 7, Medicare's financial hemorrhaging contributed to the crowding out of universal coverage in the 1980s due to the necessity of rationalizing the program's system for reimbursing hospitals. With the advent of its Prospective Payment System (PPS) in 1983, Congress switched Medicare— as the name suggests—from a retrospective to a prospective scheme of payment.[51] This major transformation had a number of unintended consequences, the most significant of which was the private sector's massive paradigm shift from fee-for-service indemnity insurance to managed care. The shift was largely an effort by employers to blunt the deleterious effects of public-to-private cost-shifting that the PPS engendered.

Table 1.1
Policy Feedback and Stages of Health Care Policymaking

Policy Feedback Type	**Failure & Frustration** (1935-early 1960s)	**Partial Success** (mid 1960s-early 1970s)	**Failure & Frustration II** (mid 1970s-present)
Interest group activity	Substantial impact: AMA dominates*	Substantial impact: labor blocks compromise plan for universal coverage in 1974	Moderate impact: "hyperpluralism" dilutes interest group influence
Policy learning	Negligible impact in the beginning, but increasing over time	Substantial impact: positive and learning effects leading to Medicare's passage*	Moderate impact: results in Medicare's PPS in 1983, managed care's growth in private sector
Lock-in effects	Initially non-existent, but gradually increasing over time	Moderate impact	Substantial impact: policymaking constrained by both locked-in policy paths and the accumulated costs of inherited programs (namely Social Security & Medicare)*
Welfare State Periods:	*Formative*	*Expansion*	*Rationalization*

* Denotes leading form of policy feedback in that stage.

By the 1990s, policy feedback reached critical mass. The traditional path of incrementally expanding existing programs was virtually defunct, but lock-in effects blocked any exit to a new path of policymaking (table 1.1). The entrenched paths of private insurance for workers and public insurance for retirees (and the poor) created a phalanx of political actors that effectively resisted the major systemic change that comprehensive reform required. Evidence of this inability to forge a new way of reaching universal coverage was provided by President Clinton's ill-fated Health Security Act of 1993-94, which vividly illustrated the futility of trying to reconcile old institutional arrangements with new policy paths. Clinton's proposal was a logical but politically flawed mix of expansion and cost containment, exposing its sponsors to the twin perils of both. In the end, path dependency rendered the politics of retrenchment politically intractable and the politics of expansion financially unaffordable.[52]

*   *   *   *

How providers deliver medical care, what its costs are, and how individuals obtain insurance coverage are political concerns of the first order. They are, as Martha Derthick observes, issues "of principle that have stirred the passions and mobilized interest groups on a massive scale."[53] The average level of public spending in OECD countries on health care is 8 percent of the gross domestic product (GDP), with the United States exceeding every other country at 15 per-cent.[54] It is all the more peculiar, then, that while the United States devotes far more wealth to health care—in absolute terms and as a percentage of GDP—than any other country, it remains the single major Western nation lacking universal coverage.

This returns us to the initial question: What explains the persistent, puzzling, and unique absence of universal coverage in the United States? The following analysis attempts to answer this question by digging into the archives that record the political motivations and struggles of individual efforts at health care reform,[55] along with, more important, their ramifications.

Notes

1. "Nixon Sees Passage in '74 of Health Insurance Plan," *New York Times*, February 6, 1974, 16.

2. "Drive for Health Bill This Session Intensifies," *Washington Post*, August 14, 1974, A8.

3. Jimmy Carter, *Public Papers of the President of the United States*, 1979 (Washington, D.C.: GPO), 1031.

4. See Roy Lubove, *The Struggle for Social Security 1900-1935* (Cambridge, Mass.: Harvard University Press, 1968), 67; and *Congressional Quarterly's Guide to U.S. Elections*, 3d ed. (Washington, D.C.: Congressional Quarterly Press Inc., 1994), 267.

5. See E. Witte, *Social Security Perspectives* (Madison: University of Wisconsin Press, 1962), 333-36, 375-77.

6. State of the Union Message (January 5, 1949), in Harry S Truman, *The Public Papers of the President of the United States, 1949* (Washington, D.C.: GPO), 5.

7. "Address before a Joint Session of the Congress on the State of the Union, January 25, 1994," *Weekly Compilation of Presidential Documents* 30 (January 31, 1994).

8. George Stephanopoulos, *All Too Human: A Political Education* (New York: Little, Brown & Co., 1999), 198.

9. Between 15 and 17 percent of the population lack health insurance coverage. See Employee Benefit Research Institute, *Sources of Health Insurance and Characteristics of the Uninsured* (Washington, D.C.: January 1994), 36-43.

10. Ellen Immergut, *Health Politics: Interest and Institutions in Western Europe* (Cambridge: Cambridge University Press, 1992), 56.

11. For more on this theory, see Louis Hartz, *The Liberal Tradition in America* (New York: Harcourt, Brace, 1955); and Sven Steinmo, "American Exceptionalism Reconsidered: Culture or Institutions," in *The Dynamics of American Politics*, ed. L. C. Dodd and C. Jillson (Boulder, Co.: Westview Press, 1994), 106-31.

12. Paul Pierson, "Increasing Returns, Path Dependence, and the Study of Politics," Program for the Study of Germany and Europe, Working Paper Series 7.7 (Center for European Studies, Harvard University, September 1, 1997), 3. See also, Paul Pierson, *Dismantling the Welfare State? Reagan, Thatcher, and the Politics of Retrenchment* (Cambridge: Cambridge University Press, 1994).

13. E. E. Schattschneider, *Politics, Pressures and the Tariff* (New York: Prentice-Hall, 1935), 288.

14. Peter Flora and Arnold J. Heidenheimer, *The Development of Welfare States in Europe and America* (London: Transaction, 1981), 292: "Once the broad Social Security Act was on the books most subsequent income maintenance and social service programs were added to it, so that . . . the most salient feature of the American welfare state is that almost all measures were passed as amendments to the original Social Security Act. The decision to overcome this bitter resistance to health insurance by also adding the Medicare and Medicaid programs in this way may well have inhibited subsequent attempts to lay the basis for a more universal health insurance program."

15. Andrew Achenbaum, *Social Security: Visions and Revisions* (Cambridge: Cambridge University Press, 1986), 167.

16. Margaret Weir, *Politics and Jobs: The Boundaries of Employment Policy in the United States* (Princeton, N.J.: Princeton University Press, 1992), 18-19. See also, K. Thelen, "Historical Institutionalism in Comparative Politics," 1998 APSA paper (Boston), 39-40; and Annual Review of Political Science 2 (1999): 369-404.

17. See John Zysman, "How Institutions Create Historically Rooted Trajectories of Growth," *Journal of Industrial and Corporate Change* 3 (November 1994): 243-83.

18. John Ikenberry, "History's Heavy Hand: Institutions and Politics of the State," paper presented at the Conference on "New Institutionalism," University of Maryland (October 14-15, 1994), 16ff.

19. See Adam Przeworski, *Capitalism and Social Democracy* (Cambridge: Cambridge University Press, 1985); and John Stephens, *The Transformation From Capitalism to Socialism* (London: Macmillan, 1979).

20. For more on this observation, see Michael Shalev, "When Markets Fail: Social Welfare in Canada and the United States," in *Welfare States in Transition*, ed. G. Esping-Anderson (London: Sage Publications, 1997), 124-25, table 5.5; Theda Skocpol, *Protecting Soldiers and Mothers: The Political Origins of Social Policy in the United States* (Cambridge, Mass.: Harvard University Press, 1992); and A. Heidenheimer, H. Heclo, and T. Adams, eds., *Comparative Public Policy* (New York: St. Martin's Press, 1990), ch. 7.

21. See Anderson 1972, Jacobs 1993, Navarro 1992, 1994, Morone 1995, Rothman 1997. Ideological or cultural theories look for explanations in the values and ideologies to which each nation's citizens adhered as urbanization and industrialization gathered forces. For more on the general theory of ideology (or culture or "national values"), see Samuel Huntington, *The Clash of Civilizations and the Remaking of World Order* (New York: Simon & Schuster, 1996); and Gaston Rimlinger, *Welfare Policy and Industrialization in Europe and America* (New York: Wiley, 1971).

22. See Alford 1975, Laham 1993, Navarro 1976, Poen 1979. Interest group theories resemble those social welfare theories (welfare capitalism and political class struggle) that focus on class conflict. The main unit of analysis is not the political system as a whole or the individuals within, but the social groups, classes, or coalitions that come into conflict. For more on the general theory of interest groups, see Peter Gourevitch, *Politics in Hard Times* (Ithaca, N.Y.: Cornell University Press, 1986); and A. Przeworski and M. Wallerstein, "The Structure of Class Conflict in Democratic Capitalist Societies," *American Political Science Review* 76 (1982): 215-38.

23. See Maioni 1995, Steinmo and Watts 1995. Institutional theories emphasize institutional relationships, both formal and conventional, that bind the components of the state together and structure its relations with society. For more on institutional theory, see Peter Hall, *Governing the Economy* (New York: Oxford University Press, 1986); J.

March and J. P. Olsen, "The New Institutionalism: Organizational Factors in Political Life," *American Political Science Review* 78 (September 1984): 734-49; and S. Steinmo, K. Thelen, and F. Longstreth, *Structuring Politics* (Cambridge: Cambridge University Press, 1992).

24. Immergut, *Health Politics*, 249, fn. 25, and xii: "[P]ublic policies should not be viewed merely as the result of the demands of various groups competing for political influence."

25. Immergut, *Health Politics*, 18.

26. Jacob S. Hacker, "The Historical Logic of National Health Insurance," *Studies in American Political Development* 12 (Spring 1998): 83: "The implication . . . about sequence and timing is that policy design matters. Political scientists generally treat public policy as the result of political processes, leaving to policy analysts the task of exploring the content of policies and their long-term effects. . . . Far from starting with a blank slate, policymakers almost always labor in the shadows of an extensive framework of existing policies that critically shapes the types of problems they perceive, the policy lessons they learn, the political conditions they face, and the types of policy instruments they have at their disposal. This is precisely why studies of policy development must take long-term historical processes into account."

27. B. Moore Jr., *Social Origins of Dictatorship and Democracy* (Harmondsworth: Penguin, 1973); T. Skocpol, *States and Social Revolutions* (Cambridge: Cambridge University Press, 1979); and P. Pierson, "When Effect Becomes Cause: Policy Feedback and Political Change," *World Politics* 45 (July 1993): 595-628.

28. Robert D. Putnam, *Making Democracy Work* (Princeton, N.J.: Princeton University Press, 1993), 8.

29. See Richard Rose and Phillip Davies, *Inheritance in Public Policy: Change without Choice in Britain* (New Haven, Conn.: Yale University Press, 1994).

30. See Bert Rockman, "The New Institutionalism and the Old Institutions," in *New Perspectives on American Politics*, ed. Lawrence C. Dodd and Calvin Jillson (Washington, D.C.: Congressional Quarterly Press Inc., 1994), 146-49: "The historical approach to the role of institutions in policy-making tends to lie outside the orbit of positivist methodologies, which seek to operationalize variables, quantify them, and formalize an explanatory structure through a process of analytic decomposition. By way of contrast, the historical approach seeks not to decompose but to recompose—to intertwine the play of societal forces with institutional structures and processes, rather than dissect them. Policy-making patterns over time suggest to us the range of feasible options for the future." For more on historical-institutionalism, see Skocpol, *Protecting Soldiers and Mothers*; and M. Weir, A. Orloff, and T. Skocpol, eds., *The Politics of Social Policy in the United States* (Princeton, N.J.: Princeton University Press, 1988).

31. See R. Bates, A. Greif, M. Levi, J. L. Rosenthal, and B. Weingast, eds., *Analytic Narratives* (Princeton, N.J.: Princeton University Press, 1999); and Margaret Levi, "Producing an Analytic Narrative," in *Critical Comparisons in Politics and Culture*, ed. John Bowen and Roger Peterson (New York: Cambridge, 2000).

32. Dietrich Rueschemeyer, Evelyne Huber Stephens, and John D. Stephens, *Capitalist Development and Democracy* (Chicago: University of Chicago Press, 1992), 387. See also, Thelen, "Historical Institutionalism in Comparative Politics," 33: These types of analyses "engage in close examination of sequences and processes as they unfold, and perhaps even more importantly, as different processes . . . unfold in relation to one another."

33. Daniel J. Goldhagen, *Hitler's Willing Executioners* (New York: Knopf, 1996).

34. Ruth Berins Collier and David Collier, *Shaping the Political Arena: Critical Junctures, the Labor Movement, and Regime Dynamics in Latin America* (Princeton, N.J.: Princeton University Press, 1991), 29-40.

35. Hacker, "The Historical Logic of National Health Insurance," 78.

36. For more on increasing returns, see Paul M. Romer, "Increasing Returns and Long-Run Growth," *Journal of Political Economy* 94 (1986): 1002-37.

37. Pierson, "Increasing Returns, Path Dependence, and the Study of Politics," Working Paper Series 7.7, 5.

38. Paul Pierson, "Increasing Returns, Path Dependence, and the Study of Politics," *American Political Science Review* 94 (June 2000): 253.

39. Pierson, "Increasing Returns, Path Dependence, and the Study of Politics," *American Political Science Review*, 253. Pierson uses a different mathematical illustration involving a Polya urn process, but the basic logic is the same.

40. Pierson, "Increasing Returns, Path Dependence, and the Study of Politics," *American Political Science Review*, 254-66. See also, Brian W. Arthur, *Increasing Returns and Path Dependence in the Economy* (Ann Arbor: University of Michigan Press, 1994).

41. For more on this dynamic of "collective action," see Mancur Olson, *The Logic of Collective Action* (Cambridge, Mass.: Harvard University Press, 1965).

42. Charles Darwin, *On the Origin of the Species* (London: Cambridge University Press, 1975).

43. See Arthur, *Increasing Returns and Path Dependence in the Economy*; Paul David, "Clio and the Economics of QWERTY," *American Economic Review* 75 (1985): 332-37; Paul Krugman, "History and Industry Location: The Case of the Manufacturing Belt," *American Economic Review* 81 (1991): 80-83; and Pierson, "Increasing Returns, Path Dependence, and the Study of Politics," Working Paper Series 7.7, 7-10: "The increasing returns variant of path dependence arguments has been applied to the development of the QWERTY typewriter keyboard, the triumph of the light-water nuclear reactor in the United States, the battles between Betamax and VHS video recorders, and DOS-based and Macintosh computers, early [car] designs, and competing standards for electric current."

44. Pierson, "Increasing Returns, Path Dependence, and the Study of Politics," Working Paper Series 7.7, 8. See also, Douglass C. North, *Institutions, Institutional Change, and Economic Performance* (New York: Cambridge University Press, 1990), 7; and Stephen Krasner, "Sovereignty: An Institutional Perspective," *Comparative Political Studies* 21 (April 1988): 66-94.

45. Policy elites also played an important role in crafting the proposed legislation for old age insurance (OAI).

46. See Arthur F. McClure, *The Truman Administration and the Problems of Postwar Labor, 1945-48* (Rutherford, N.J.: Fairleigh Dickinson Press, 1969); Harold W. Metz, *Labor Policy of the Federal Government* (Washington, D.C.: The Brookings Institution, 1945); and Harry A. Millis and Emily Clark Brown, *From the Wagner Act to Taft-Hartley: A Study of National Labor Policy and Labor Relations* (Chicago: University of Chicago Press, 1950).

47. For more on the theory of incrementalism, see Richard Rose and B. Guy Peters, *The Juggernaut of Incrementalism: A Comparative Perspective on the Growth of Public Policy* (Glasgow: University of Strathclyde, 1978); and M. Hayes, *Incrementalism and Public Policy* (New York: Longman, 1992).

48. For more on opportunity windows and the related issue of agenda setting, see John Kingdon, *Agendas, Alternatives, and Public Policies* (New York: HarperCollins,

1984), 173-80; Frank R. Baumgartner and Bryan D. Jones, *Agendas and Instability in American Politics* (Chicago: University of Chicago Press, 1993); and Gary Mucciaroni, *Reversals of Fortune: Public Policy and Private Interests* (Washington, D.C.: The Brookings Institution, 1995).

49. For elaboration on this point, see Martha Derthick, *Policymaking for Social Security* (Washington, D.C.: The Brookings Institution, 1979), 316-38.

50. Robert Ball, "Medicare's Roots: What Medicare's Architects Had in Mind," *Generations* 20 (Summer 1996): 13.

51. Prior to 1983, with relatively few limits Medicare retrospectively paid the charges that doctors and hospitals submitted for treating patients. After 1983, Medicare paid doctors and hospitals a predetermined figure for treating patients. If the predetermined figure was more or less than the actual cost of treating the patient, the medical provider pocketed the difference or absorbed the loss, respectively.

52. For more on this issue, see Pierson, *Dismantling the Welfare State?*

53. Derthick, *Policymaking for Social Security,* 337.

54. Organization for Economic Cooperation and Development (OECD), *The Reform of Health Care Systems* (Paris: OECD, 1994), 37-39; and OECD, "Economic Surveys" (Paris: OECD, 1996-98).

55. For more on this style of approach, see Immergut, *Health Politics,* 54-58.

CHAPTER TWO

Critical Juncture

Health Insurance Subordinated to Social Security
(1935)

Social Security is a cornerstone which is being built, but is by no means complete—a structure intended to lessen the force of possible future depressions, to act as a protection to future administrations of the government against the necessity of going deeply into debt to furnish relief to the needy—in other words, a law that will take care of human needs and at the same time provide for the United States an economic structure of vastly greater soundness.

—President Franklin D. Roosevelt,
Signing of the Social Security Act (August 14, 1935)

Speaking before a country mired in the Great Depression, President Roosevelt triumphantly announced the inauguration of Social Security.[1] It was a plan that had hitherto been politically infeasible—a relatively comprehensive and potentially universal[2] national welfare program. Frances Perkins, Roosevelt's secretary of labor and chair of the Committee on Economic Security (the group charged with drafting the social security bill), recorded in her memoirs that policymakers desired three "principal items" of social protection at the time: "unemployment insurance, about which we had come to definite views; old-age insurance, which looked more difficult; and health insurance."[3] Roosevelt shared these goals, as Jaap Kooijman has documented, but with regard to the third—health insurance—he was skeptical of its passage and concerned that including it would imperil the enactment of the rest of the act.[4] Consequently, when Franklin D. Roosevelt signed Social Security into law in 1935, health insurance was the only protection of the three excluded. This omission ignited a quest for the passage of a health insurance program that would wax and wane for the rest of the century.

17

A number of questions serve to guide this chapter. What explains the different political outcomes of old age insurance and health insurance? Why was illness the only threat to loss of income that was excluded from Social Security? Essential in addressing the main question of this study, what were the political and developmental consequences of old age insurance and health insurance being sent off on different trajectories?

Although a health insurance program did not pass during Roosevelt's presidency, the period is significant because it constitutes the welfare state's most important "critical juncture." Critical junctures are leading determinants of how programs and policymaking develop, with outcomes during a crucial transition establishing distinct pathways or trajectories of growth.[5] Formidable political legacies ordinarily emerge after critical junctures as a product of the continuity and equilibrium that return following these "great spurts" of change.[6] "What all critical junctures have in common is their fundamental impact on subsequent historical dynamics," observes Jacob Hacker. "The ways in which crucial periods of transition occur shape processes of political and economic development for decades to come."[7] The passage of the Social Security Act is an excellent example.

An examination of the events surrounding the critical juncture of Social Security's passage illustrates the two crucial pathways of policymaking that emerged. These pathways, public for old age insurance and (eventually) private for health insurance, predestined many of the combatants, issues, and arguably many of the outcomes of political battles for the decades that followed. Most important, the exclusion of health insurance from the Social Security program created a critical relationship between old age insurance (OAI) and health insurance. A public program for the latter became dependent on the former.

Social Security as a Critical Juncture: Inclusion and Exclusion

Americans today take Social Security for granted as an institution of immense economic and political influence. In the early 1930s, however, the term did not exist. Instead, policymakers focused on welfare in the first year of Roosevelt's administration, engaging in a flurry of activities designed to alleviate the immediate scourges of unemployment and economic stagnation. These efforts constituted the First New Deal.

By 1934, Roosevelt was ready to turn his administration's attention toward longer-term changes in the economic landscape. Concerned that his early programs such as the NRA (National Recovery Administration) and AAA (Agricultural Adjustment Administration) would disappear once economic growth returned, he wanted to leave a more permanent legacy that could not be dismantled. Social Security became the embodiment of Roosevelt's desire. As the welfare state's biggest critical juncture of the century, it started the Second New Deal.

As the vehicle for the drafting of Social Security, Roosevelt created the Committee on Economic Security (CES) by Executive Order 6757 on June 29,

1934. The committee consisted of several members of the president's cabinet.[8] Many social insurance experts from academia and government joined the CES as staff members, including Professor Edwin E. Witte of the University of Wisconsin as the committee's director. Although many CES staff members desired a cradle-to-grave system of social insurance, political exigencies made it impossible. Social Security would incorporate some protections, but not all of them.

Dramatic departures in public policy are rare,[9] but the severity of the Depression in the early 1930s fostered a demand for action on the part of the national government. Roosevelt's creation of the CES represented a rare instance in which the policymakers involved were more "choosers" than "heirs."[10] Economic calamity produced a chance for policy departure and innovation. Members of the CES took advantage of this "window of opportunity"[11] to introduce new and ambitious social insurance programs.

Rather than inheriting national public policies, Roosevelt commissioned the committee's members to draft largely new ones. Most of their policy-making experience in social insurance, if they had any, came from state initiatives in workmen's compensation. Their work was constrained on one side by the perceived constitutional and administrative limits that existed, and pressured on the other side by the expressed demands of highly mobilized political movements in the form of "Townsendism" and Huey Long's "Share the Wealth" campaign. These movements do not fit the precise description of interest groups, as we know the term today, but as social movements they produced a dynamic that contributed crucially to the pressure for Congress to act.

AMA Dominates Health Insurance Policymaking

Until programs and institutions are in place, interest groups and policy elites tend to dominate the shaping of public policies.[12] By 1934, these sets of actors were familiar with the political characteristics of public health insurance, which had been debated since the issue of compulsory health insurance first arose in the latter part of the first decade of the twentieth century.[13] A few individual state legislatures, notably those in California and New York, had briefly considered statewide health insurance plans in the late 1920s as possible companions to their fledgling workmen's compensation programs. Their goal was to form a total package of worker-related protection. Physicians, represented by AMA, ultimately crystallized their opposition to the states' proposals in a resolution unanimously endorsed at an AMA House of Delegates convention in 1922:

> The American Medical Association hereby declares its opposition to all forms of "state medicine," because of the ultimate harm that would come thereby to the public health through such form of medical practice.
> "State medicine" is hereby defined for the purpose of this resolution to be any form of medical treatment, provided, conducted, controlled, or subsidized by the federal or any state government.[14]

The AMA operated as an effective interest group with narrow but clearly enunciated goals.[15] It anticipated that the CES would suggest some form of health insurance, and reacted immediately when it did.[16] At the National Conference on Economic Security, held in November 1934 to elicit public support for the CES's proposals, the AMA launched its attack. Two prominent physicians—whom CES leaders expected to endorse the desirability of health insurance—changed their position without prior notice and attacked pro-insurance members of the CES's subcommittee: the Medical Advisory Committee (MAC). According to CES Executive Director Witte, the MAC became a lightning rod for controversy over the proposed inclusion of health insurance:

> The list of members of the Medical Advisory Committee was carried in the newspapers of the first Sunday of November [1934]. Before the midnight of that day, scores of telegrams had poured in upon the President, principally from physicians. . . . [They] protested the alleged unfairness of the Committee on Economic Security and its staff. Literally hundreds of telegrams of this vein were sent to the President or to members of the committee.[17]

Leaders of the CES came to believe that health insurance would be defeated in Congress, due to the AMA's opposition.[18] Worse, they feared that an attempt to include it might imperil the passage of the entire Social Security proposal.[19] In Daniel Hirshfield's opinion, "The medical society's opposition was a powerful force which could be turned against unemployment and old age legislation, and they wanted to avoid this contingency at all costs."[20] At best, according to Paul Starr,

> some members of the Committee on Economic Security and its staff thought that Congress would act quickly on unemployment and old-age programs and that health insurance could be introduced later in the same session. This expectation proved to be mistaken. Even a discussion of general principles for health insurance in the committee's January report aroused a storm of protest from the AMA. These principles included assurances that private medical practice would continue; that the medical profession would control professional personnel and procedures; and that doctors would be free to choose their patients, the method of reimbursement, and whether to participate in insurance practice.[21]

Deterred by the AMA's opposition, Edwin Witte wrote that—because of the AMA's opposition—he and President Roosevelt came to the opinion that the inclusion of health insurance "was politically impossible . . . and would spell defeat for the entire bill."[22]

Roosevelt was sympathetic to health insurance, but he and members of his staff were also acutely conscious of the vehement opposition to its inclusion.[23] The president wanted Congress to give the old age and unemployment programs top priority. In his message to Congress on January 17, 1935, calling for passage of legislation that was later to become the Social Security Act, Roosevelt omitted any call for a health insurance program, stating (somewhat disingenuously): "I am not at this time recommending the adoption of so-called 'health insurance,' although groups representing the medical profession are cooperating with the federal government in the further study of the subject and definite progress is being made."[24] Congress should consider a health insurance program, he felt, only if it were noncontroversial (which, of course, was impossible).[25] Many years later, Roosevelt publicly revealed his fear of the AMA. Discussing the issue of health insurance with a key Senate committee chairman in 1943, Roosevelt said, "We can't go up against the State Medical Societies; we just can't do it."[26] His previous experience as governor of New York had convinced him of organized medicine's formidable strength.

Besides, Congress had no desire to pursue a public health insurance scheme. "Indeed, the strength of the anti-insurance feeling in Congress [was] illustrated by the action taken by the House Ways and Means Committee to delete the words 'health insurance' from the list of topics on which the bill authorized the Social Security Board to conduct research," notes Hirshfield. "Signs of the strength of anti-insurance sentiment in Congress continued to grow and apparently convinced the President that the whole issue was too politically explosive to keep in open view."[27] Thus, by June 1935 the AMA's Reference Committee on Legislative Activities confidently reported that it had been in contact with President Roosevelt's Committee on Economic Security and had gained the strong impression "that compulsory sickness insurance would not be presented at this, nor very likely at the next session of Congress."[28]

Administrative Aspects of Health Insurance Increase AMA's Effectiveness

Roosevelt was dissuaded not only for political reasons but also for logistical ones. "Hospital construction was one of the obvious needs of the time, because there were so many communities that had no good hospital and there was great debate within our committee [the CES] as to where hospitals should be placed and what was a minimum size hospital that would be able to provide even general medical care," recalls Dr. Martha Eliot, assistant chief of the Children's Bureau.[29] The president and others believed that if a health insurance program ever were to be administratively feasible, there would have to be many more hospitals. "Roosevelt had been impressed with the need for hospital service in many parts of the country," wrote CES Chair and Labor Secretary Frances Perkins, "and [he] saw this as a substitute for health insurance."[30]

The bureaucratic implications of old age insurance and health insurance increased the effectiveness of the AMA's opposition to the Social Security Act including health insurance. As Ellen Immergut has noted:

> The involvement of the medical profession is in fact what makes national health insurance so controversial. In this area of social policy, governments do not merely provide transfer payments [as with public pensions]; they pay for the services of a private profession that is highly organized and politically influential. From the perspective of governments, such an open-ended commit-

ment is problematic. Whereas the costs of pensions, for example, can be predicted, the costs of national health insurance depend upon the costs of medical treatment. These costs are potentially limitless, for they increase as doctors experiment with new therapies, patients demand new treatments, and the charges for medical procedures go up. Indeed, opponents of national health insurance have often argued that this is a Pandora's box of never-ending costs.[31]

The different administrative demands required of old age insurance and health insurance worked to the advantage of the former and to the distinct disadvantage of the latter.

Two structural aspects proved to be politically critical: (1) third-party providers, and (2) actuarial predictability. The first, third party providers,[32] made health insurance far more difficult to pass than old age insurance. Old age insurance did not need, nor did it arouse opposition from, any intermediary or third-party provider. As the interest group equivalent to the medical profession, the private insurance industry was consciously apolitical. It was unwilling to jeopardize its tradition of generating enormous profits by attracting increased government attention and possible regulation. Martha Derthick explains, "Whether in regard to social security or any other subject, the [private insurance] industry was reluctant to take a conspicuous part in national politics. . . . The industry's great size and wealth made it an inviting target of government inquiry."[33]

The private insurance industry could be ignored and, thus, bypassed by Congress and Roosevelt in a way that the medical profession (as represented by the AMA) never could. Old age insurance only threatened an inconsequential percentage of the private insurance industry's market share: its old age annuities. National health insurance, on the other hand, posed a dramatic threat to the prevailing cash-based or out-of-pocket method of paying for medical care. The structure of OAI afforded the private insurance industry the legitimate option of remaining politically agnostic. Organized medicine did not perceive itself to have the same luxury. Finally, the popularity of old age insurance's closely related, means-tested cousin, old age assistance (OAA), helped to insulate OAI behind the tidal wave of support it created.[34]

Unlike old age insurance, health insurance required a third-party provider: doctors at least and hospitals, arguably. As previously discussed, these groups were the leading political force in strident opposition to any inclusion of health insurance. Those who would have had to cooperate for a health care program to work flatly refused to do so. The AMA swore that it would never tolerate the intrusion of government into its private affairs regardless of how flexible and lucrative the remuneration scheme might be.

The second factor that made old age insurance much easier to pass than health insurance was actuarial predictability. In other words, because old age insurance specifically targeted those age sixty-five and older, actuarial estimates of the program's costs could be made with some semblance of credibility. The structure of old age insurance delineated a system of routine contributions over a specified period of time that generated a determinable level of benefits to begin at a mutually agreed upon date. Nevertheless, actuarial estimates of old age insurance still faced difficulties, because policymakers had to make assumptions based on circumstances that would change over decades (rate of economic growth, birth rate, mortality rate, and so forth).

But if old age insurance had some actuarial and administrative challenges, those of health insurance were greater by several magnitudes. Conceivably, its constituency could be young working adults, the retired elderly, or both. Not only were the demographics of the constituency nearly impossible to predict, so was the level of benefits. An individual might or might not incur physician and hospital expenses in a given year. Would health insurance cover both or just one? If just one, which one and why? Would there be a cost-sharing component (e.g., a deductible or copayment) whereby individuals would need to cover a portion of the costs? If so, how would these figures be determined? If an individual required medical care, the costs could range from minor to catastrophic. Actuarial predictions would be enormously difficult to make.

Roosevelt's own lack of confidence, together with the controversy surrounding health insurance, led him to exclude the subject from the CES's final report.[35] He never even publicly released the CES's separate report on health insurance. Instead, he secretly transmitted it to the Social Security Board in January 1936, requesting that "the Board undertake such research as part of its program during the balance of the present fiscal year and, if necessary, during the succeeding fiscal year."[36]

Thus, the president's Social Security proposal to Congress contained just one oblique reference to health insurance as a subject that the new Social Security Board should study. But as Executive Director Witte observed, "that little line was responsible for so many telegrams to the members of Congress that the entire Social Security program seemed endangered until the Ways and Means Committee unanimously struck it out of the bill."[37]

Huey Long and Townsendism: Catalyst for Congressional Action

In contrast to the AMA's effective campaign against health insurance, Huey Long's "Share the Wealth" campaign and Townsendism played influential roles in producing pressure *for* Congress to pass something (albeit in the end not to either group's liking). Mobilized in response to the new political and economic incentives presented, the leaders of these movements were eager to obtain any redistributive advantage that new government policies might provide. Their main interest was not Roosevelt's proposed Social Security scheme, but more radical measures.

Huey Long considered Roosevelt's proposals too timid and insufficient to remedy the pernicious effects of the Depression. Instead, his "Share the Wealth" campaign called for a minimum level of provision for housing, food, and income, along with a maximum level of annual income for an individual (approximately $1 million). The government would confiscate any income above this level and redistribute it to the public. Long's assassination in September 1935, however, abruptly ended the organized structure of his "Share the Wealth" movement and its political strength in mobilizing public opinion.[38]

The second and more significant interest group movement took the form of Townsendism. During the establishment of the CES in the summer of 1934—while Long was reaching his peak of influence—Dr. Francis Townsend was known more to social insurance experts, such as the CES's Wilbur Cohen, than to the general public. None of his future interest group's 7,000 clubs or 3.5 million members were yet organized. But by the end of 1935, Dr. Townsend's movement had become the greatest catalyst for the administration's Social Security plan. The core tenets of Townsendism competed against Social Security's old age insurance until as late as the early 1950s.[39] Essentially, the movement called for the distribution of $200 each month by the federal government to every citizen over the age of sixty-five. The revenue would come from taxes on "the entire American community." The organization's plan made the benefits contingent on a recipient's immediate retirement and pledge that all of the money would be spent by the end of each month.

Guided by an intuitive Keynesianism,[40] Townsendism was far more radical than Social Security. Most experts derided the group's demands, considering them to be a potential disaster. The reaction of most congressmen ranged from scorn to abject fear: "Townsendism is the most extraordinary social and political movement in recent years and perhaps in our entire history," lamented Senator William E. Borah.[41] Claude Pepper, a Democratic senator from Florida at the time, agreed, but he also pointed to the role of Townsendism in propelling Social Security:

> It went through changes in its form, but the agitation for the Townsend Plan had a lot to do with the expansion of the Social Security concept and the Social Security program. I've said many times that Dr. Townsend and Franklin Delano Roosevelt together deserved a large part of the credit for the adoption and the expansion of the Social Security program.
>
> *Q. Dr. [Arthur] Altmeyer agrees, that the 1939 amendments in particular were due to Townsend pressure.*
>
> That's right. [Townsendism] got weaker as the years went on and the Social Security system improved, but undoubtedly it had a considerable influence in the improvement of the system.[42]

While highlighting the plight of the elderly and thrusting this formidable constituency into the political arena, Townsendism specified a proposal that was unrealistic. The more Congress and the public examined its plan, the more dubious its remedies appeared. Nevertheless, Townsendism contributed to the congressional acceptance of an alternative: old age insurance that the CES devised and Roosevelt proposed.[43] "The effect Townsendism created," wrote CES Executive Director Witte, "was that the real issue became the Townsend plan or Social Security."[44] Roosevelt agreed: "We have to have it. The Congress can't stand the pressure of the Townsend Plan unless we have a real old-age insurance system."[45] Thus, the Townsend plan and Huey Long's "Share the Wealth" proposal helped Social Security, because they created the political pressure that forced Congress to pass something on behalf of the elderly and unemployed.

Conclusion

Roosevelt subordinated health insurance to old age insurance in 1935 primarily so that Social Security could be passed. As a critical juncture, Social Security's passage left health insurance in a position both secondary to and, in time, dependent on OAI. The main hindrance to a national health insurance program was the AMA's interest group opposition. Of the three programs proposed for inclusion in the Social Security Bill, only health insurance generated such intense opposition.[46] Moreover, the administrative necessities of health insurance greatly disadvantaged its prospects for inclusion and passage.

By comparison, old age insurance was much more feasible to implement. Old age insurance passed mostly because old age assistance (OAA) carried it. A much more popular program, OAA had no opposition and a tremendous amount of support. For many in Congress, OAI also became an attractive alternative to the more radical measures of Townsendism and Huey Long's "Share the Wealth" campaign. The choice in 1935, then, was to start down a public path for old age insurance and to reject a public path for health insurance. Roosevelt's decision to exclude health insurance proved to be crucial; the first, relatively comprehensive and potentially universal welfare-state program in the United States began without health insurance.

Notes

1. The term *Social Security* is semantically problematic. Most individuals currently view Social Security as synonymous primarily, if not exclusively, with government old age pensions (OASI). The term actually comprises all the programs taxed for by the FICA (Federal Insurance Contributory Act) payroll deduction: old age, survivors, dependents, and disability insurance, and Medicare. All these programs, however, were not what was initially included in the original eleven titles of the Social Security Act passed in 1935: Title I, Old Age Assistance (OAA); Title II, Old Age Insurance (OAI); Title III, Unemployment Compensation; Title IV, Aid to Dependent Children (ADC); Title V, Family Health Grants; Title VI, Public Health Service; Title VII, Social Security Board; Title VIII, Financing for OAI; Title IX, Financing for Unemployment Compensation; Title X, Aid to Needy, Blind, and Disabled; and Title XI, Terms and Administration.

2. Frances Perkins, *The Roosevelt I Knew* (New York: The Viking Press, 1946), 282-83: "At cabinet meetings and when [Roosevelt] talked privately with a group of us, he would say, 'There is no reason why everybody in the United States should not be cov-

ered. I see no reason why every child, from the day he is born, shouldn't be a member of the social security system. When he grows up, he should know he will have old-age benefits direct from the insurance system to which he will belong all his life. If he is out of work, he gets a benefit. If he is sick or crippled, he gets a benefit. . . . Everybody ought to be in on it. . . . Cradle to the grave-from the cradle to the grave they ought to be in a social insurance system'. . . a universal approach."

3. Perkins, *The Roosevelt I Knew*, 289.

4. See J. Kooijman, "Soon or Later On: Franklin D. Roosevelt and National Health Insurance, 1933-1945," *Presidential Studies Quarterly* 29 (June 1999): 336.

5. Paul David, "Clio and the Economics of QWERTY," *American Economic Review* 75 (May 1985): 332.

6. Ruth Berins Collier and David Collier, *Shaping the Political Arena: Critical Junctures, the Labor Movement, and Regime Dynamics in Latin America* (Princeton, N.J.: Princeton University Press, 1991), 28-29. See also, Max Weber, ed., *On Charisma and Institution Building* (Chicago: University of Chicago Press, 1968), 1111.

7. Jacob Hacker, "The Historical Logic of National Health Insurance," *Studies in American Political Development* 12 (Spring 1998): 78.

8. Frances Perkins, labor secretary (chair); Henry Morgenthau, treasury secretary; Homer Cummings, attorney general; Henry Wallace, agriculture secretary; and Harry Hopkins, federal emergency relief administrator.

9. Richard Rose and Phillip Davies, *Inheritance in Public Policy: Change without Choice in Britain* (New Haven, Conn.: Yale University Press, 1994), 1.

10. Rose and Davies, *Inheritance in Public Policy*, 1. As Rose and Davies maintain, "policymakers are usually heirs rather than choosers."

11. See John Kingdon, *Agendas, Alternatives, and Public Policies* (New York: HarperCollins, 1984).

12. See Paul Pierson, *Dismantling the Welfare State: Reagan, Thatcher, and the Politics of Retrenchment* (Cambridge: Cambridge University Press, 1994), 40; and Theda Skocpol, *Protecting Soldiers and Mothers: The Political Origins of Social Policy in the United States* (Cambridge, Mass.: Harvard University Press, 1992).

13. See Ronald L. Numbers, *Almost Persuaded: American Physicians and Compulsory Health Insurance, 1912-1920* (Baltimore, Md.: Johns Hopkins University Press, 1978); and J. Dennis Chase, "The American Association for Labor Legislation and the Institutionalist Tradition in National Health Insurance," *Journal of Economic Issues* 28 (December 1994): 1063-90.

14. *Journal of the American Medical Association* 78 (Chicago: American Medical Association, April 1922): 1715.

15. See James Rorty, *American Medicine Mobilizes* (New York: W. W. Norton, 1939).

16. See Howard Wolinsky and Tom Brune, *The Serpent on the Staff* (New York: G. P. Putnam, 1994), 20-21.

17. Edwin Witte, *The Development of the Social Security Act* (Madison: University of Wisconsin Press, 1962), 174-77.

18. Paul Starr, *The Social Transformation of American Medicine* (New York: Basic Books, 1982), 267: "From the outset the prevailing sentiment on the Committee on Economic Security was that health insurance would have to wait. Edwin Witte, the staff director, recorded in a confidential memo in 1936 his 'original belief that medical society opposition precluded any action on health insurance.' This view was shared by Secretary Perkins. Harry Hopkins, the relief administrator, was 'more interested in health insurance than in any other phase of social insurance, but also realized that this subject would have

to be handled very gingerly.' Nor was this sentiment confined to members of the committee. In an article published in October of 1934, Abraham Epstein, the founder of the American Association for Social Security and a leading figure in the movement, advised the administration to be politically realistic and specifically to go slow on health insurance because of the opposition it would arouse—this from someone who later would become severely critical of the conservatism of the Social Security bill."

19. Interview with Martha Eliot, Oral History Collection, Columbia University (1965): "Concerning the debate over health insurance, I sat as an observer in some of the Committee meetings, and I can remember the anxiety on the faces of the members of that Committee, on both sides of the game." (Hereafter Eliot, OHC.)

20. Daniel S. Hirshfield, *The Lost Reform: The Campaign for Compulsory Health Insurance in the United States from 1932 to 1943* (Cambridge, Mass.: Harvard University Press, 1970), 57: "In order to protect those programs to which they gave the highest priority, these senior members of the CES evolved a policy which could legitimately delay or ultimately suppress the publication of the pro-insurance Final Report of the Technical Committee on Medical Care."

21. Starr, *The Social Transformation of American Medicine*, 268: "Without definitively recommending a plan, the committee listed as goals the provision of adequate medical services, the budgeting of wage losses and medical costs, 'reasonably adequate remuneration' to practitioners, and new incentives for improved medical care. The system the committee envisioned was to be state administered, and state participation would be optional. The role of the federal government was to provide subsidies and set minimum standards for states that adopted a health insurance program. As the reformers now generally agreed, cash benefits in sickness would be separate, probably linked with unemployment insurance."

22. Witte, *The Development of the Social Security Act*, 188. See also, Theron Schlabach, *Edwin E. Witte: Cautious Reformer* (Madison, Wis.: State Historical Society of Wisconsin, 1969), 112-14; Michael M. Davis, *Medical Care for Tomorrow* (New York: Harper and Bros., 1955), 277; Rashi Fein, *Medical Care, Medical Costs* (Cambridge: Cambridge University Press, 1986), 42; and Richard Carter, *The Doctor Business* (New York: Doubleday & Co., Inc., 1961), 199-200.

23. Thomas Eliot, *Recollections of the New Deal* (Boston: Northeastern University Press, 1992), 111: "I was thankful that the Committee on Economic Security had decided to leave health insurance out of the bill. Its inclusion would have aroused such vehement opposition, sparked by the American Medical Association, that the whole bill, even the simple grants to the states, would have gone down the drain. . . . In 1935 even sacrificing health insurance did not ensure passage of a bill that included other forms of social insurance."

24. *Journal of the American Medical Association* 91 (Chicago: American Medical Association, March 1935): 749. See also, Elton Rayack, *Professional Power and American Medicine: The Economics of the American Medical Profession* (New York: The World Publishing Company, 1967), 167.

25. Interview with Arthur Altmeyer, Oral History Collection, Columbia University (1965), 28-33. (Hereafter Altmeyer, OHC.)

26. John M. Blum, *From the Morgenthau Diaries: Years of War* (Boston: Houghton Mifflin, 1967), 72. See also, Starr, *The Social Transformation of American Medicine*, 279.

27. Hirshfield, *The Lost Reform*, 60. See also, Witte, *The Development of the Social Security Act*, 188-89; and Starr, *The Social Transformation of American Medicine*, 268.

28. *Journal of the American Medical Association* 91 (Chicago: American Medical Association, June 1935): 2366. See also, Rayack, *Professional Power and American Medicine*, 170.

29. Eliot, OHC, 81.

30. Perkins, *The Roosevelt I Knew*, 297. See also, "Roosevelt Plans to Build Hospitals for Needy Regions," *New York Times*, December 23, 1939, 1.

31. Ellen Immergut, *Health Politics* (Cambridge: Cambridge University Press, 1992), 12. See also, William A. Glaser, *Paying the Doctor under National Health Insurance: Foreign Lessons for the United States* (Springfield, Va.: National Technical Information Service, U.S. Department of Commerce, 1976).

32. Examples could include insurance companies, doctors, hospitals, or other benefit providers.

33. Martha Derthick, *Policymaking for Social Security* (Washington, D.C.: The Brookings Institution, 1979), 140: "Measured by its assets, the Metropolitan Life Insurance Company was the biggest business in the country in 1937, though it subsequently gave way to another insurance company, the Prudential Insurance Company of America. In 1972, both exceeded the assets of Standard Oil of New Jersey and General Motors, their nearest rivals, by more than $10 billion. For such behemoths to pursue an aggressively self-interested course was a considerable risk to public relations, and it has been a point of pride with insurance company executives that they did not spend big money in national politics in contrast, say, to the petroleum or dairy industries [or organized medicine]."

34. OAA consisted of flat-rate monthly stipends to any senior citizen poor enough to qualify for the program. For more information on OAA, see Derthick, *Policymaking for Social Security*, 217-22, 273-74.

35. Hirshfield, *The Lost Reform*, 58-59; and Witte, *The Development of the Social Security Act*, 187-89. The committee's full report is included as Appendix III in Witte's memoir, 205-10: "Letter of Transmittal and Summary of Major Recommendations on Health Insurance from the Committee on Economic Security to the President" (November 6, 1935).

36. Arthur Altmeyer, *The Formative Years of Social Security* (Madison, Wis.: University of Wisconsin Press, 1966), 58.

37. Witte, *The Development of the Social Security Act*, 182-83; Interdepartmental Committee to Coordinate Health and Welfare Activities, The Nation's Health (Washington, D.C.: GPO, 1939), 103.

38. The definitive work on Huey Long is T. Harry Williams's *Huey Long* (New York: Knopf, 1969).

39. The definitive work on Townsendism is Abraham Holtzman's *The Townsend Movement: A Political Study* (New York: Bookman Associates, 1963).

40. Townsendism focused on stimulating the demand for goods by increasing the public's overall purchasing power, while ostensibly opening up jobs for younger workers, all in an effort to perk up the economy.

41. Witte, *The Development of the Social Security Act*, 86.

42. Interview with Claude Pepper, Oral History Collection, Columbia University (1968), 14.

43. *The Gallup Public Opinion Poll, 1935-1971* (New York: Random House, 1972), 9. Public opinion agreed with the Townsend movement's demand that something be done on behalf of the impoverished elderly, but it did not agree with Townsendism: 89 percent favored government old age pensions for needy persons, yet only 4 percent of the country favored the Townsend plan, while 96 percent opposed it.

44. Witte, *The Development of the Social Security Act*, 86.
45. Perkins, *The Roosevelt I Knew*, 294.
46. Roosevelt chose, instead, to pursue the goal of increased hospital construction.

CHAPTER THREE

Diverging Pathways

The Aftermath of Social Security's Passage
(mid-1930s to early 1950s)

A national health insurance program will soon be legislated, because the Democrats are going back in power, and we are going to see that we get it.

—President Harry S Truman (1948)

The decade and a half following the critical juncture of Social Security's passage marked a period of slow growth for the public path of old age insurance (OAI), while the AMA continued to dominate the issue of health insurance. Policymakers were consumed with creating Social Security's administrative infrastructure and protecting the program from its enemies. During this time, OAI remained in the shadow of its more popular and larger welfare competitor, old age assistance (OAA). Social insurance enthusiasts strongly disliked OAA, in part because it was not a contributory entitlement program upon which they could build other insurance protections (as OAI was). But they were in no position to dismantle the program. Meanwhile, in a parallel effort, advocates of health insurance pursued the passage of a national health insurance program. Their ambitions translated into omnibus proposals of legislation that opponents, particularly the AMA, found easy to defeat. In one reprise of the original 1935 decision after another, a public path for health insurance was rejected during this period.

Social Security and OAI's Struggle for Survival

Old age insurance grew slowly in the first year following its passage.[1] The Social Security Act set taxation for financing the OAI trust fund to begin in 1937, and benefits to commence even later in 1942. In addition, old age insurance was only for industrial and commercial workers, covering barely 50 percent of the employed workforce.

31

Notable exclusions from OAI included: farm labor, domestic service, casual labor, maritime employment, the self-employed, the publicly employed, and nonprofit organizations. It would take the remainder of 1935 and all of 1936 just to construct the administrative capacity to run a program of Social Security's magnitude in an age when computers existed exclusively in the realm of science fiction.

With the public path of OAI barely begun, the program was vulnerable to criticism, particularly in regard to its funding. Policymakers designed old age insurance to be self-financing through a payroll tax. Roosevelt wanted a program that would not be dependent on general revenues. With taxes scheduled to begin in 1937, benefits in 1942, and contributors far outnumbering beneficiaries, estimates predicted that a trust fund surplus would eventually mushroom to a staggering $47 billion by 1980. The figure was eight times the amount of money in circulation in 1937 and twice the government debt.[2] The Republican presidential nominee, Alf M. Landon, assailed Social Security in the 1936 election as "unjust, unworkable, stupidly drafted, wastefully financed, and a cruel hoax."[3] Landon was overwhelmingly defeated, but criticism of the program did not end with the 1936 election.

Reacting to an initiative by Republican Senator Arthur Vandenberg to look into the problem of a massive surplus, Congress created the second Advisory Council on Social Security (the first came in 1935). Part of the council's recommendation to solve the surplus problem included benefits starting in 1940 instead of 1942, and for benefits to be larger than originally proposed. The council also suggested that OAI should seek to collect taxes from new groups of employees by absorbing many into the program who were originally excluded.[4]

The advisory council of 1937-38 shifted the emphasis of the OAI program from equity to adequacy[5] (e.g., adding monthly benefits to workers' spouses and, in the event of deaths, their survivors and dependents). In other words, the focus became the protection of the family unit rather than solely an individual.[6] Robert Ball, chief executive of the SSA from 1962 to 1973, argues that "the 1937-38 council was probably the most important of all the advisory councils in determining the original understanding and the continuing shape of the Social Security program. The entire history of Old Age, Survivors, and Disability Insurance (OASDI) from 1939 to the amendments of 1972 can be described as rounding out the structure recommended by this council."[7]

Without realizing how dramatic and significant the council's recommendations for change were, Congress passed them as the Social Security Amendments of 1939.[8] Ironically, conservative criticism of the system's financing led to measures that ultimately put the program on a path to significantly greater expansion. With benefits arriving two years earlier than planned and the addition of dependents and survivors, the new OASI adjusted the policy balance in favor of "social adequacy."[9]

In producing such a fundamental change in Social Security's coverage, the 1939 amendments reinforced OASI's public pathway of development and growth. In other words, the amendments bolstered social insurance as a permanent *public* institution. Congress abandoned the intention of creating a large trust fund, and changed the system to a cash basis or a pay-as-you-go system.[10] Two years before his death, Wilbur Cohen (the second "Mr. Social Security" after his mentor, Arthur Altmeyer) provided a candid account of the 1939 amendments compiled from his direct observations:

> The importance of the 1939 amendments is that they came so quickly after the 1935 Act, which no one could have predicted. . . . Now what we didn't know at that time is that the war was going to break out, and what happened in effect was that you had a major, tremendously significant reform of social security. It was not viewed that way then because it was slightly before benefits came out and because it satisfied [Senator Arthur] Vandenberg that the New Deal wouldn't be spending all this money in the future on reckless items. So it wasn't viewed as if it was a big reform; it was viewed as a reaffirmation and a continuation [of the original scheme]. But it broadened the benefits immediately and got the system started in an atmosphere of bipartisan support.
>
> In my opinion, the 1935 Act, the 1937 constitutionality ruling, the 1939 amendments, the war coming out—all these together meant that when social security was up for reexamination in 1949 and 1950—the issue of changing the system . . . never had any reality.[11]

Cohen's quote illustrates the importance of the 1939 amendments. While thinking that they had succeeded in limiting Social Security's growth, the program's opponents actually expanded it and helped to secure its existence. On the last day of the decade (December 31, 1939), the *New York Times* entitled one of its articles "Era of Social Security Begins for the Worker: Pension Payments to Those over 65 to Start Next Month in a Great Federal Test of Paternalism."[12]

AMA Dominates Health Insurance Debate

Meanwhile, social insurance advocates began their efforts for a public health insurance program immediately after its exclusion from Social Security. As the Committee on Economic Security had argued, "No national program of economic security can be regarded in any sense as complete or effective without adequate provision for meeting the risks to security which arise out of ill health."[13] Roosevelt responded by establishing an Interdepartmental Committee to Coordinate Health and Welfare Activities. The committee began by simply considering the coordination of existing health activities, but early in 1937 it turned to the broader question of developing a national program of medical care. Arthur Altmeyer, chairman of the SSB and a leading member of the committee, was largely responsible for this change in the committee's direction. It was done, he claims, with Roosevelt's approval, but not his explicit support.[14]

A subsidiary group to Roosevelt's interdepartmental operation, the Technical Committee on Medical Care, quickly emerged to deal with a program of health insurance. The Social Security Board's I. S. Falk guided what the subgroup considered and, ultimately, proposed. The fruit of the Technical Committee's labors was a proposal in February 1938 entitled "National Health Program." The program had five basic components, the fourth of which was clearly the most controversial:

1) Expansion of existing federal public, maternal and child health services.
2) Expansion of national hospital facilities through federal grants.
3) Federal assistance to state medical care systems for the medically needy.
4) A general program of medical care, paid for either through general taxation or social insurance contributions.
5) Establishment of federally assisted disability insurance to provide cash payments for temporary loss of wages.[15]

Recognizing the wrath that the fourth recommendation would arouse from organized medicine (AMA), the committee assigned it the lowest priority and couched it in the least specific terms.[16]

Seeking to publicize the program's agenda and build momentum for health insurance, Roosevelt announced a "National Health Conference" to be held in Washington in July 1938. In response, the AMA called a special session and agreed to support all of the program's recommendations except number four, which advocated universal coverage. The AMA tried to make a deal with Roosevelt that it would openly support four of the program's five recommendations if he agreed to drop the proposal for a national health program. The president refused. According to Altmeyer, Roosevelt was so encouraged by the success of the conference that he seriously considered making the National Health Program an issue in the upcoming off-year congressional elections. Then, without apparent reason, he decided to postpone any effort until the 1940 presidential campaign. Altmeyer intimates that he may have wanted to use the issue in his pursuit of a third term in office.[17]

Despite opposition from the AMA, Republicans, insurance executives, and "states righters," as well as Roosevelt's lack of support, Senator Robert Wagner of New York proceeded with health insurance legislation. Wagner incorporated most of the National Health Program's five recommendations into a bill proposed in 1939 that, if passed, would have included amendments to the original Social Security Act and become the "National Health Act."[18] Social insurance advocates had already given some consideration to adding health insurance to the 1939 Social Security amendments. But Arthur Altmeyer, chairman of the Social Security Board, recalls that everyone involved understood that health insurance was still an extremely controversial and sensitive issue: "Just as in 1935, it was felt unwise [in 1939] to jeopardize more basic and more important priority items by attaching a controversial issue like health insurance. So it was decided to keep it as a separate but parallel effort."[19]

The AMA responded to Wagner by stating that it would offer no opposition to health insurance as long as it was voluntary.[20] Senator Wagner did make his plan voluntary, by watering it down into a *federal* health insurance plan consisting of grants to those states that opted to participate.[21] But Roosevelt still refused to publicly support the plan, referring to it as a "grandiose scheme," and instead urged that more hospitals be built.[22] Wagner's bill, S. 1620, received perfunctory hearings but never got out of committee due to disagreement over what constituted sufficient "medical need."[23] With the onset of World War II, and the massive rearmament that absorbed America's attention, public health insurance slowly died as "an orphan of the New Deal."[24]

A Public Path for Health Insurance Repeatedly Frustrated

The 1940s continued the feeling of frustration for proponents of universal health insurance coverage. Those who favored nationalizing health insurance to varying degrees encountered insuperable resistance from private interests. Equally discouraging, the political battles over a public program for medical care were chaotic, characterized by a dizzying number of competing plans.

National health insurance advocates sought to capitalize on the rapidly increasing cost of medical care in the early 1940s, which enraged patients and created a public demand for government to make health care more affordable. By August 1943, 60 percent of the public favored expanding Social Security to include payment of benefits for sickness, disability, doctor, and hospital bills. Only 29 percent were opposed, with the rest undecided.[25] Equally encouraging to social insurance enthusiasts was that 75 percent of those who claimed to be in favor of adding benefits to Social Security for medical costs also reported that they were in favor of paying an additional 6 percent of their wages in order to finance the benefits.[26]

Once implemented, a technique such as social insurance tends to be readopted, to be considered the "natural" policy response for other types of income risk.[27] The Social Security Board reacted in a similar way in the 1940s to the public's frustration with rapidly increasing medical costs. It envisioned a comprehensive scheme of insurance (similar to Britain's revolutionary Beveridge plan)[28] that would be added to the original Social Security Act. The final product of this initiative was the omnibus 1943 Wagner-Murray-Dingell Bill. It proposed to "cover the major economic hazards of the average American throughout his lifetime, such as loss of income through unemployment, illness, temporary or permanent disability, old age, medical care, and hospital services."[29] The Wagner-Murray-Dingell Bill was an American cradle-to-grave proposal. Its degree of centralized social provision, however, was exceeded only by its political impracticality.

The Social Security Board's role in drafting the 1943 Wagner-Murray-Dingell Bill was a harbinger of things to come. It anticipated the freelance style in which several SSB leaders and supporters of Social Security, above all organized labor, would come to operate in advancing their expansionist goals for health insurance. In June 1943, without Roosevelt's support, Senator Wagner introduced the first Wagner-Murray-Dingell Bill in Congress. According to Alanson Willcox, general counsel for the Social Security Board's parent, the Federal Security Agency, "Wagner-Murray-Dingell was originally and almost exclusively drafted by the Social Security Board."[30]

As before, the vehement opposition of the AMA was an insurmountable political obstacle. No hearings were ever held on the Wagner-Murray-Dingell Bill, and it died in committee. As Martha Derthick claims, though, the bill's defeat helped to educate Social Security executives in the ways of incrementalism, a strategy that would develop considerable momentum and effectiveness in the years to come:

> The Wagner-Murray-Dingell bill of 1943 . . . did not pass, or come close to being passed as a whole. Only by being broken up and considered piece by piece over many years, and with individual pieces tailored to fit political circumstances of the moment, did much of the Wagner-Murray-Dingell bill ultimately become law. A philosophy perhaps, incrementalism was also a lesson learned from experience.[31]

The SSB's Wilbur Cohen admitted later that incrementalism was, indeed, the strategy that eventually emerged: "When, in my youthful impatience I asked the Senator [Wagner] if he was going to look at the [SSB's] bill or the draft statement . . . he said no; he said it would take a number of years before the bill would ever be enacted—it would be re-drafted innumerable times and his role was to introduce it so that future members of Congress could carry it forward to realization after he was gone."[32] Wagner reintroduced the Wagner-Murray-Dingell Bill in 1945 and 1947, but, as he predicted, it failed to make any progress. Organized medicine proved too formidable an opponent.

Truman's Last New Deal Attempt at National Health Insurance

The nation's most powerful political actor, the president, had been missing from every effort for national health insurance prior to 1945. Harry Truman, however, made his support of a national health insurance program clear from the beginning of his presidency. On November 19, 1945, he delivered the first presidential message ever devoted exclusively to health care.[33] His speech made four specific recommendations:

1) Establishment of a nationwide system of health insurance.
2) Federal aid for medical education.
3) Increased federal aid for the construction of hospitals.
4) Increased federal aid for public health and maternal & child health services.[34]

Congress's enthusiasm for these recommendations was noticeably less than Truman's. Despite the president's ambition for congressional action, only piecemeal legislation passed in the following years: grants for hospital construction (the Hill-Burton Act of 1946), increased federal funding for medical research (specifically for the National Institutes of Health, NIH) and public health services. Numerous factors prevented serious consideration of Truman's full proposal. The mid-term elections of 1946 delayed any possible expansion by government in the area of health insurance, as Republicans gained majorities in both the House and the Senate. Truman's necessary campaigning for reelection in 1948 postponed more concerted efforts to make health insurance a top priority on the political agenda. The issue seemed to be losing ground.

The president's upset victory, though, together with the defeat of many Republicans of the "Do-Nothing" Congress in 1948, led political observers to believe—as Arthur Altmeyer suggests—that 1949 would finally witness the passage of a public health insurance program:

> *Q. When he won that upset victory, one had the impression that after that, Truman felt he had a mandate for all kinds of things.*
>
> (Altmeyer): That's right. There was a period of a few months there [after Truman's victory] where light seemed to have blazed again from the firmament and all was going to be wonderful.[35]

Following his reelection, Truman reiterated his call for Congress to enact a compulsory health insurance program in his State of the Union address on January 5, 1949. He was the first president to use this annual address to the nation to demand national health insurance: "In a nation as rich as ours, it is a shocking fact that tens of millions lack adequate medical care," he exclaimed. "We need—and we must have without further delay—a system of prepaid medical insurance."[36] Truman repeated his demands a few days later in his Economic Report, his Annual Budget Message, and in a Special Message to the Congress on the Nation's Health Needs in April of the same year.[37] Once in Congress, his initiative became the fourth Wagner-Murray-Dingell Bill. Despite the optimism of Truman and his supporters, however, the giant presence of the AMA loomed over the entire debate.

The AMA's Opposition

The American Medical Association continued to dominate interest-group activity in the health policy arena, as had been the case since the issue of universal health insurance first arose. This was critical, because interest group activity, in turn, dominated the political debate. Organized medicine perceived any health insurance program attached to Social Security to be a "wedge" for later incremental expansion and possible takeover of medical care by government.

Publicly, the AMA continued to argue that governmental involvement risked damaging the high quality of American health care. Privately, it based its decision on the organization's desire to maintain professional sovereignty and autonomy. For these reasons, the AMA proceeded to wage the single greatest public relations counteroffensive against Truman's proposal that the country had ever witnessed over the issue of health care policy. After raising a "war chest" by collecting $25 from every physician who was a member, the AMA hired the husband and wife public relations team of Clem Whitaker and Leone Baxter, now considered to be the first modern-day political consultants. Over the course of its campaign against the attachment of a universal health insurance program to Social Security, the AMA spent the then-unprecedented sum of nearly $5 million.[38] As Paul Starr explains, the AMA was able to capitalize, with its use of the term "socialized medicine," on the political conditions surrounding the Cold War:

> "Would socialized medicine lead to socialization of other phases of American life?" asked one pamphlet, and it answered, "Lenin thought so. He declared: 'Socialized medicine is the keystone to the arch of the Socialist State'." (The Library of Congress could not locate this quotation in Lenin's writings.) So successful was the campaign in linking health insurance with socialism that even people who supported Truman's plan identified it as "socialized medicine," despite the administration's insistence it was not. Support in public opinion polls, among those who had heard of Truman's plan, dropped from 58 to 36 percent by 1949; three quarters of those who had heard of the plan knew of the AMA's opposition. As anticommunist sentiment rose in the late forties, national health insurance became vanishingly improbable.[39]

Much to social insurance advocates' dismay, the AMA's dominance was enhanced by the technical or administrative problems associated with Truman's proposal. Similar to the flaws that politically disadvantaged the original Wagner-Murray-Dingell bills, Truman's proposed legislation did not specify clearly how much revenue would be necessary and how expenditures would be distributed. Would doctors be directly reimbursed or would individuals who needed medical care simply receive cash benefits to cover their costs? Would the SSA use corporate intermediaries to process payments? How would the states be involved, if at all? Neither Truman's 1949 bill nor the earlier Wagner-Murray-Dingell versions addressed these fundamental questions, conceded Alanson Willcox, the Social Security Administration's general counsel:

> I remember generally that [the proposals] seemed to us awfully fuzzy in many places. It wasn't at all clear what was intended. The material, I think, was not very well organized. The methods of administration were far from clear. . . . There was a lot of confusion about the qualifications, as I remember it, of participants in providing services. . . . I remember we felt the bill was not as good a job as could be done by any means. Senator Murray, who had become the chief protagonist on the Hill, recognized this partly I think as the result of criticisms that were made. He came to realize that a better job could be done.[40]

The vagueness of Truman's plan weakened its political prospects, thereby amplifying the AMA's effectiveness. But the organizational makeup of Congress made them even more unpromising. Lacking an institutionalized routine for considering competing health insurance plans, Congress was unable to constrain the free flow of participants and the plans they could propose. A proliferation of alternative health insurance proposals resulted. For instance, financier Bernard Baruch recommended a national system of voluntary health insurance for high-income Americans and compulsory insurance under Social Security for low-income people.[41] Senators Ralph Flanders and Irving Ives and Congressman

Richard Nixon called for a locally controlled, government-subsidized, private nonprofit insurance system, with premiums scaled to subscribers' incomes.[42] Senators Lister Hill and George Aiken proposed a program calling for the government to provide federal assistance to the states to subsidize premium payments for the poor on private plans such as Blue Cross.[43] Finally, Senators Robert Taft, Forrest Donnell, and H. Alexander Smith reintroduced an earlier version of their plan to offer a medical welfare system for the nation's indigent that would be financed through federal grants and administered entirely by participating states.[44] Draining political loyalty to any one plan, the increased number of alternatives to Truman's plan decreased the likelihood that any one of them could pass.

This unrestrained atmosphere in Congress enhanced the effectiveness of the AMA's opposition. Truman's 1949 bill became so contentious that the institutional process for deliberation in Congress gradually ground to a halt. The Bill never made it out of committee.[45] Although the president had a sizable partisan majority in both houses of Congress, he and his fellow supporters were far from securing a programmatic majority. Moreover, Social Security was not yet popular, so trying to add a health insurance program to it did not resonate with the public or Congress.

Truman later recalled, "I have had some bitter disappointments as President, but the one that has troubled me most, in a personal way, has been the failure to defeat organized opposition to a national compulsory health insurance program."[46] The leaders of the New Deal, who succeeded in establishing various social welfare initiatives, did not and could not provide the necessary political means for policymakers to pass a public health insurance program. The AMA's victory secured health insurance's exclusion from any public path.

OASI's Contrasting Fortune: The 1950 Social Security Amendments

At the start of 1940, there were 9,100,000 Americans age sixty-five and over, none of whom were receiving OASI benefits, while 2,170,000 were OAA beneficiaries. As late as 1949, OAA's monthly cash payments were 70 percent larger than those of OASI.[47] With health insurance stalled in the 1940s, explains Katherine Ellickson of the CIO, social insurance advocates shifted their attention to Social Security's OASI program:

> [I]t was clear that the political situation was not such that there was any real hope of getting health insurance through . . . , because the war was taking the primary efforts of the country, and then when the war was over, there were obvious improvements that were needed in old age and survivors' insurance which had not been enacted, and so the first push was for something about that. And of course that wasn't politically possible until 1950.[48]

The unions' shift from focusing on health insurance to OASI coincided with Congress's growing belief that it would eventually have to make a choice between it and OAA. In their efforts to protect OASI, executive leaders of the newly renamed Social Security Administration (formerly Social Security Board) approached the Republican-led Congress in 1947 to ask for a new advisory council.

The 1947-48 council came out strongly in favor of OASI. It exposed the great disparities existent between agricultural and industrial states when it came to the issue of OAA benefits for the elderly: "Because employers and employees paid for social insurance but welfare came partly out of a state or county's general revenues, poorer agricultural states faced greater financial burdens in aiding the elderly than did richer industrial states."[49] The council's findings and recommendations favored the championing of OASI through changes that would increase the generosity of its benefits and the number of beneficiaries.

Figure 3.1
OAA and OASDI Beneficiaries as a Percentage
of the Population Aged Sixty-Five and Over, 1940-80*

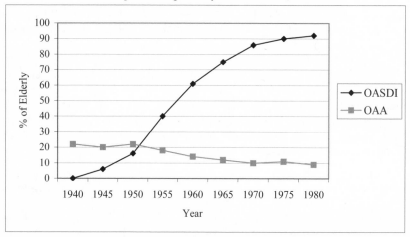

Source: Adapted from U.S. Department of Health and Human Services, Social Security Administration, *Social Security Bulletin, Annual Statistical Supplement, 1985*, 235.
* Old Age Assistance (OAA) became subsumed under Supplemental Security Income (SSI) in 1974.

It is no surprise, then, that Congress eventually accepted the council's recommendations and opted for OASI. Whereas the amendments of 1939 settled the issue of Social Security's financing, the second set of amendments in 1950 settled the contest between welfare and insurance (figure 3.1). The 1950 amendments extended OASI coverage to groups formerly excluded, such as farm, domestic, and self-employed workers. They also boosted benefits for OASI beneficiaries equal to those of old age assistance. The result was that OASI benefits increased immediately by 77 percent, and many more people began receiving benefits sooner than originally planned.[50]

The 1950 amendments bolstered OASI's increasing political and economic returns, in large part because they radically increased the program's revenues. In turn, increased revenues translated into bigger benefits for many more people, which substantially enlarged the program's popularity. As OASI's generosity and number of beneficiaries grew, employers gradually incorporated the program's bigger benefits into the private pension arrangements that they annually negotiated with labor unions.

Old age and survivors insurance was on solid footing by the century's halfway point, the most secure it had been since its inception. The contest with OAA and its means-tested structure was over and OASI had won.

Conclusion

Social Security's passage in 1935 initiated a public pathway for old age insurance, but precluded one for health insurance. Nevertheless, organized labor and SSA leaders continued to pursue health insurance as a separate, parallel effort. They hoped to replicate the success of Social Security by enacting a public health insurance program to complement OASI. Their repeated failures were due mostly to the formidable interest group opposition of organized medicine, as represented by the AMA. In contrast to Social Security's OASI, deliberation over health insurance was marked by a vehement partisanship and ideological confrontation. Instead of narrowing, as they did for OASI, health insurance measures proliferated whenever Congress addressed the issue. The still minimal amount of policy feedback from either policy learning or lock-in effects during this period left interest group activity—and, thus, the AMA—in a position of dominance.

The divergence between the two policy areas continued in keeping with the original outcome of Social Security's passage in 1935. Policymakers secured OASI's public path, while their attempts at forging a similar path for health insurance failed repeatedly. Congress's solidifying of OAI with the 1939 and 1950 amendments institutionalized the program, and made it ready for exponential growth and expansion in the decades to follow.

Notes

1. A Gallup poll in November of 1936 reported 68 percent in favor of the compulsory old age insurance plan that was set to start in January of 1937, and 32 percent opposed. *The Gallup Public Opinion Poll, 1935-71* (New York: Random House, 1972), 40.

2. Arthur Altmeyer, *The Formative Years of Social Security* (Madison: University of Wisconsin Press, 1966), 88-89.

3. *Vital Speeches of the Day* 3 (New York: The City News, October 15, 1936), 26.

4. Altmeyer, *The Formative Years of Social Security*, 89-93.

5. For further explanation, see Martha Derthick, *Policymaking for Social Security* (Washington, D.C.: The Brookings Institution, 1979), 213-27.

6. J. Douglas Brown, *An American Philosophy of Social Security* (Princeton, N.J.: Princeton University Press, 1972), 136.

7. Robert Ball, "The Original Understanding on Social Security," in *Social Security: Beyond the Rhetoric of Crisis*, ed. Theodore Marmor and Jerry Mashaw (Princeton, N.J.: Princeton University Press, 1988), 25.

8. Interview with Arthur Altmeyer, Oral History Collection, Columbia University (1965), 65 (hereafter Altmeyer OHC): "So the upshot was that we got the proposal to Congress in 1939 to improve the benefits, start them sooner, include the survivors' benefits and dependents' benefits as well as the primary beneficiaries'. The effect was—and I made a point of that—to cut down the size of the reserve by paying out more money in the early years and less money in the later years. I used the illustration of a seesaw to indicate the curve of benefit payment instead of going up steeply like that would start at a higher level and go up less steeply. The net result would be a system that would not cost any more but would use up the reserve enough in the early years to keep it from building up to an unconscionable level."

9. Robert J. Myers, *Social Insurance and Allied Government* (Homewood, Ill.: R. D. Irwin, 1965), 6: "Whenever a social security system involves contributions from the potential beneficiaries, the question of individual equity versus social adequacy arises. Individual equity means that the contributor receives benefits protection directly related to the amount of his contributions—or, in other words, actuarially equivalent thereto. Social adequacy means that the benefits paid will provide for all contributors a certain standard of living. The two concepts are thus generally in direct conflict, and social security systems usually have a benefits basis falling between complete individual equity and complete social adequacy. Usually, the tendency is more toward social adequacy than individual equity." See also, J. Pechman, H. J. Aaron, and M. K. Taussig, *Social Security: Perspectives for Reform* (Washington, D.C.: The Brookings Institution, 1968), 33-34.

10. Myers, *Social Insurance and Allied Government*, 6.

11. Cohen quoted in *Social Security: The First Half-Century*, ed. Gerald Nash, Noel Pugach, and Richard Tomasson (Albuquerque: University of New Mexico Press, 1988), 79-82.

12. *New York Times*, December 31, 1939, 10: "On New Year's Day the Federal Government's answer to the Townsend plan and all the other fantastic programs which have sprung from the depression will become effective. On that day the first old-age benefits will be payable under the liberalized Social Security Act, the most comprehensive experiment in paternalism in history, and before the end of the month, the first checks will have been mailed."

13. See Committee on Economic Security, *Social Security in America* (Washington, D.C.: GPO, 1937).

14. Altmeyer, *The Formative Years of Social Security*, 93-95.

15. United States Interdepartmental Committee to Coordinate Health and Welfare Activities, *Proceedings of the National Health Conference* (Washington, D.C.: GPO, 1939), 29-32.

16. Altmeyer, *The Formative Years of Social Security*, 95-96.

17. Altmeyer, OHC, 117: "Roosevelt was so impressed that I remember very distinctly he said, 'We'll make that an issue this fall in the campaigns.' That was an off-year. But he no more than said that before he said, 'No, I think it would be better to wait for a Presidential year,' which would have been '40. Whether he was thinking of running

in 1940 for a third term, I don't know, and whether he thought this would be a vote-getter, I don't know. But he didn't think it was just the right time to shoot the works."

18. "National Health Program Offered by Wagner," *New York Times*, March 1, 1939, 1; and "Wagner's Health Bill Result of Long Drive," *New York Times*, March 5, 1939, Part IV.

19. Altmeyer, OHC, 110.

20. "Health Insurance Favored by Millions," *New York Times*, January 22, 1939, 9.

21. S. 1620, 76th Congress, 1st Session; "National Health Bill," *New York Times*, March 12, 1939, Part IV.

22. "AMA Chief Fishbein Praises Hospital Program," *New York Times*, December 31, 1939, 21.

23. "The Health Hearings," *New York Times*, June 11, 1939, Part IV, editorial, 8.

24. Theodore Marmor, *The Politics of Medicare* (Chicago: Aldine, 1973), 9. Altmeyer, OHC, 117: "Of course by the time 1939 rolled around, World War II had started and Roosevelt was completely involved in that from the very beginning. All this domestic reform became secondary."

25. *The Gallup Public Opinion Poll*, 1935-1971, 400.

26. *The Gallup Public Opinion Poll*, 1935-1971, 400.

27. Hugh Heclo, *Modern Social Politics in Britain and Sweden* (New Haven, Conn.: Yale University Press, 1974), 305.

28. Britain's "Beveridge Plan" called for a national, contributory system of social insurance that would cover such contingencies as ill health, unemployment, permanent disability, old age, and the need for medical care. It was financed by contributions from a worker, the employer, and the government. The Beveridge Plan was a blueprint for a cradle-to-grave system of social insurance many in the SSB viewed with envy. Roosevelt was envious, if not also faintly jealous: "When Roosevelt read the reports of the Beveridge Plan he jokingly said to me one day, 'Frances, what does this mean? Why does Beveridge get his name on this? Why does he get credit for this? You know I have been talking about cradle-to-grave insurance ever since we first thought of it. It is my idea. It is not the Beveridge Plan. It is the Roosevelt Plan'" (Frances Perkins, *The Roosevelt I Knew* [New York: Viking Press, 1946], 283).

29. Poen, *Harry S. Truman versus the Medical Lobby*, 32: "Included were provisions for the payment of unemployment compensation to returning veterans while they looked for jobs; for the nationalization of both the United States Employment Service and the country's unemployment insurance system; for increased old-age social security payments; for the addition of millions of temporary and permanently disabled workers to the benefit rolls; for liberalization of federal aid in support of state welfare systems; and, most important, for the creation of a comprehensive, government-directed prepaid medical-care program. . . . Doctors' [fees would be] paid—subject to a rate limitation imposed by the government—through a fund established and maintained by payroll taxes. If hospital services became necessary, national health insurance would underwrite a patient's expenses for up to sixty days of confinement per year. Significantly, the Wagner-Murray-Dingell bill centralized postwar responsibility for economic welfare. Whereas Wagner's 1939 proposal had envisaged state-operated health and welfare services, his 1943 manifesto called for federal sponsorship and direction." See also, S. 1161 and H.R. 2861, 78th Congress, 1st Session.

30. Interview with Alanson Willcox, Oral History Collection, Columbia University (1965), 13.

31. Derthick, *Policymaking for Social Security*, 26.

32. Wilbur Cohen, "From Medicare to National Health Insurance," in *Toward New Human Rights: The Social Policies of the Kennedy and Johnson Administrations*, ed. David C. Warner (Austin: The University of Texas, Lyndon B. Johnson School of Public Affairs, 1977), 144.

33. "A National Health Program: Message from the President," *Social Security Bulletin* (December 1945).

34. Altmeyer, *The Formative Years of Social Security*, 171. See also, Harry S Truman, *Years of Trial and Hope, 1946-1953* (New York: Doubleday, 1956), 22.

35. Altmeyer, OHC, 138.

36. State of the Union Message (January 5, 1949), in Harry S. Truman, *The Public Papers of the Presidents of the United States, 1949* (Washington, D.C.: GPO), 5.

37. Poen, *Harry S. Truman versus the Medical Lobby*, 26, 27, 226-30.

38. Howard Wolinsky and Tom Brune, *The Serpent on the Staff* (New York: G. P. Putnam, 1994), 23-25.

39. Paul Starr, *The Social Transformation of American Medicine* (New York: Basic Books, 1982), 285.

40. Interview with Alanson Willcox, Oral History Collection, Columbia University (1967), 17.

41. Poen, *Harry S. Truman versus the Medical Lobby*, 227.

42. S. 1970, H.R. 4924, 81st Congress, 1st Session.

43. S. 1581, S. 1456, 81st Congress, 1st Session.

44. S. 545, 81st Congress, 1st Session; and Altmeyer, *The Formative Years of Social Security*, 171.

45. *New York Times*, 27 October 1949.

46. Truman, *Years of Trial and Hope*, 25.

47. Marmor and Mashaw, *Social Security: Beyond the Rhetoric of Crisis*, 28; and Derthick, *Policymaking for Social Security*, 273.

48. Interview with Katherine Ellickson, Oral History Collection, Columbia University (1966), 15.

49. Edward D. Berkowitz, *America's Welfare State from Roosevelt to Reagan* (Baltimore, Md.: Johns Hopkins University Press, 1991), 58.

50. Ball, "The Original Understanding on Social Security," 31.

CHAPTER FOUR

Increasing Returns

Institutionalization of Public and Private Pathways
(early 1950s through early 1960s)

It would appear logical to build upon the system [Social Security] that has been in effect for almost twenty years rather than embark upon the radical course of turning it upside down and running the very real danger that we would end up with no system at all.

—President Dwight D. Eisenhower
to investment banker E. F. Hutton (1953)

As with so many other parts of the American society and economy in the post-war years, Social Security and private health insurance experienced tremendous growth. A confluence of steady economic prosperity, a rising birth rate, and virtual full employment provided the perfect conditions for their institutionalization. In 1950, Social Security's old age and survivors insurance program (OASI) covered just 16 percent of the population. A decade later political leaders had increased the figure to 60 percent.[1] Likewise, in 1948 only 8 percent of all Americans had comprehensive private health insurance (hospital and physicians' services). By 1957 the proportion had tripled to 24 percent, with 60 percent of the population in possession of at least hospital insurance.[2]

Two events less than twelve months apart precipitated this extraordinary growth in private health insurance and Social Security. In 1949 a second critical juncture in the area of medical care occurred: the ascendance of private health insurance. Labor unions caused the rapid growth of private health insurance by seeking it through collective bargaining (or group contracting) with employers on behalf of workers.[3] For Social Security, 1950 proved to be the turning point for the program's success and popularity. The Social Security amendments of that year greatly enlarged the size of OASI's benefits and its number of beneficiaries.

45

Collective bargaining for private insurance and the 1950 Social Security amendments independently laid the foundations for a series of "increasing returns." Over time, these returns made private health insurance and OASI more attractive for many more people. Paul Pierson defines increasing returns as the high fixed costs, learning and coordination effects, and adaptive expectations that come with a new policy or program.[4] Simply put, individuals make commitments based on the incentives of existing arrangements, so the cost of changing them rises dramatically over time.[5] Once Congress passed Social Security, there were strong incentives for it to keep moving down that path because greater numbers of people came to depend on the program when they retired.[6] And the incentives were magnified after 1950.

The same effect was true regarding health insurance. After organized labor realized that the American Medical Association would keep national health insurance from passing, it chose another route—insurance through collective bargaining with employers—and stuck with it after it proved effective. Increasing returns pushed individual behavior onto paths that were hard to reverse.[7]

In examining the consequences of the growth of Social Security and private health insurance during this period, there are a couple of questions to answer. If private health insurance flourished in the 1950s through collective bargaining, why did policymakers eventually begin to look to Social Security to provide some measure of protection against the cost of illness? More generally, what were the implications of Social Security's growing popularity and administrative simplicity for the future possibility of attaining universal coverage?

Private Path: The Meteoric Rise of Health Insurance

Ironically, the spark that ignited the massive increase in private health insurance was a failure—that of President Truman's ambitious national health insurance proposal in 1949. The prospects for national health insurance evaporated. But Truman's defeat happened to come soon after the National Labor Relations Board ruled that compulsory collective bargaining could include health insurance as a fringe benefit.[8] This ruling was enormously important, because under the Wagner and Taft-Hartley Acts fringe benefits were considered tax-exempt.[9]

Thus, two events were key. First, the NLRB's ruling opened the way for health insurance to be added to collective bargaining (while at the same time granting it a tax advantage). Second, Truman's defeat left organized labor with little choice but to turn to collective bargaining, which it did with enthusiasm. Alanson Willcox maintains that labor's decision "was perhaps the most influential factor in postponing, for an indefinite time, any possibility of a general national health insurance system, because it did give a tremendous fillip to voluntary health insurance."[10] James Brindle, a leader of the United Auto Workers (UAW), confirms Willcox's claim:

Some of the labor people were beginning to despair of getting a national health program. . . . It must have been in the late 1940's, when the [unions] decided: 'Let's go flat out to get voluntary health insurance without denying the need for a national system. We can't wait. We're not getting it.' They threw this in as an important item into collective bargaining by auto and steel and a whole bunch of other industrial unions first. It was almost universally the thing that sparked the tremendous expansion of voluntary health insurance.[11]

The Supreme Court confirmed the NLRB's ruling the next year in its *Inland Steel* case, which stated that benefit plans that included health insurance came within "conditions of employment."[12] Organized labor now had the right and employers had the obligation to at least negotiate over health insurance as a fringe benefit.[13] The unions' switch to collective bargaining coincided with a national campaign launched by the AMA to show that voluntary health insurance was the American way. "For the first time," Paul Starr notes, "the AMA was actually promoting health insurance."[14]

Figure 4.1
Union Membership as a Percentage of the Nonagricultural Labor Force, 1930-85

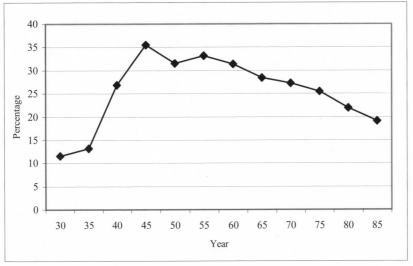

Source: T. Kochan, H. Katz, and R. McKersie, *The Transformation of American Industrial Relations* (Ithaca, N.Y.: ILR Press, 1994), 31, figure 2.1.

The effectiveness of organized labor's switch to pursuing private health insurance as a fringe benefit through collective bargaining was enhanced by a substantial increase in both union membership and unions' negotiating prowess.[15] During the late 1940s and 1950s, union membership as a percentage of the labor force peaked (figure 4.1). Between 1940 and 1954, the number of union members almost doubled, from 8,717,000 to 17,022,000.[16]

The generous 1948 General Motors (GM)-UAW agreement emerged as the model for others that followed in many industries.[17] Even in firms with no union presence, the threat of unionization induced managers to provide benefits such as health insurance to prevent demands for unionization.[18] For these reasons, among others, labors bargaining position in industrial relations during the 1950s was arguably the strongest that it has ever been.

In 1948, only 2.7 million workers had private health insurance negotiated by their unions. By 1950, the number had more than doubled to 7 million. By 1954, 12 million workers—together with their 17 million dependents—had health insurance as a result of unions' bargaining with employers, for a total of 29 million individuals.[19]

Figure 4.2
Percentage of the Population in Private Health and Pension Plans, 1942-62

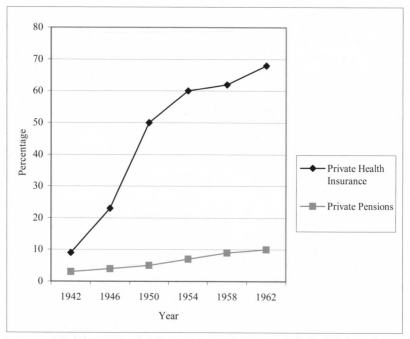

Source: Adapted and modified from Jacob Hacker and Paul Pierson, "Business Power and
        Social Policy: Employers and the Formation of the American Welfare State," paper
        presented at the American Political Science Association Annual Meeting (Washington,
        D.C.: 2000), figure 2.

The proportion of Americans with some type of health coverage, mostly hospital insurance, skyrocketed from 10 percent in 1940 to slightly more than 60 percent by 1957 (figure 4.2 provides a comparison with private pensions).[20] In turn, private insurance began to pay for a larger percentage of the nation's medical care (table 4.1). Annual premium payments—shared to varying degrees by employers and employees—soared from $100 million to $4.2 billion, a rate of growth, 25 percent per year compounded, never before witnessed in the insurance industry.[21] It is not surprising then, as Marie Gottschalk has discovered, that "the myth of the consensus years of labor-management relations in the 1950s obscures how contested an issue benefits remained at the bargaining table."[22]

Table 4.1
Private Expenditures for Medical Care in Millions and
Percentage Accounted for by Private Health Insurance, 1948-57

Year	Hospital Services Amount	Hospital Services Percentage	Physicians' Services Amount	Physicians' Services Percentage	Hospital and Physicians' Services Amount	Hospital and Physicians' Services Percentage
1948	$1,667	27.3	$2,360	6.4	$4,027	15.0
1949	1,779	30.3	2,371	9.6	4,150	18.5
1950	2,100	32.4	2,462	12.7	4,562	21.7
1951	2,289	39.2	2,556	17.8	4,845	27.9
1952	2,534	42.4	2,702	19.6	5,236	30.6
1953	2,822	45.1	2,890	22.4	5,572	33.6
1954	3,056	47.2	3,162	23.3	6,218	35.0
1955	3,383	49.6	3,242	26.4	6,625	38.3
1956	3,765	53.7	3,548	28.0	7,313	41.2
1957	4,019	57.3	3,783	30.8	7,802	44.5

Source: Agnes W. Brewster, "Voluntary Health Insurance and Medical Care Expenditures: A Ten-Year Review," *Social Security Bulletin* 21, no. 12 (December 1958): 13.

Problems with Private Health Insurance

Society's great leap to private health insurance coverage was not without its problems.[23] In some respects, private health insurance became a victim of its own success. Having helped to increase access to medical care for millions of Americans, it heightened the sense of inequity for the less privileged. Hiding behind the phenomenal growth in private program enrollment was a growing number of financial flaws and gaps in individual insurance policies. Families with insurance found themselves with uncovered expenses, forcing them to pay out-of-pocket.[24]

Even nonprofit insurance giants such as Blue Cross/Blue Shield began to experience severe financial hardship. Their tradition of "community rating" led to many of their profitable customers leaving for the corporate insurance companies that offered cheaper premiums through their use of "experience rating."[25] Finally, the growth of private insurance fed a massive rise in medical inflation (table 4.2), which posed serious problems for those on low or fixed incomes—the elderly, poor, disabled, and unemployed.

Table 4.2
Consumer Price Index: All Items and Medical Care, 1940-64*

CPI	1940	1945	1950	1955	1960	1961	1962	1963	1964
All items (inflation)	60	77	103	115	127	128	129	131	133
Hospital charges^	50	64	115	165	223	240	257	273	287
Physician charges	75	88	104	123	145	149	153	157	161
All health care	73	83	106	128	156	161	165	169	173

Source: "Expenditures for Health and Medical Care," *Progress in Health Services* (January -
      February 1963): 1-6.
* 1947-1949=100
^ per day

Another limitation of private insurance was that it rarely extended to retired workers. The unions, therefore, desired to find a way of taking care of their members after they retired.[26] If Social Security supplemented the unions' pensions, could it not do the same for their health insurance plans? These kinds of questions made Social Security an object of growing interest for those concerned with the problems of private health insurance.

The Eisenhower administration after 1953 concluded that something would have to be done to remedy private insurance's shortcomings. It did not, however, support social insurance. As Allen Pond notes, administration officials felt that "if they could get over the next five to ten years, politically speaking, and increase coverage to a very substantial proportion of the population," then social insurance could be avoided.[27] Eisenhower's administration studiously tried to prevent a "pressure valve" effect from developing, according to Beth Stevens, in which chronic problems in the private sector lead to demands for public sector solutions:

> The establishment of a welfare program by one sector . . . reduces the pressure
> on the other sector to satisfy certain needs. The establishment of Social Secu-
> rity relieved private corporations of the responsibility for providing pensions
> for poorly paid workers, and the development of private health insurance re-
> duced the pressure for national health insurance. In such a process inaction, not
> just action, is critical. The failure of one sector to develop a program increases
> pressure on the other sector because neglected groups turn to the alternative
> program.[28]

The president and his supporters were convinced that the way to avoid a pressure valve effect with health insurance was to step in and assist the private sector with its problems.

Eisenhower and conservative Republicans chose to pursue a substantial stimulation of private health insurance.[29] Some proposals included offering public funds to corporate insurance carriers as "reinsurance" in exchange for their willingness to cover pools of high-risk, uninsured individuals.[30] Other voluntary plans consisted of adjusting personal income tax policy by "either deducting from gross income the cost of insurance premiums, or providing some kind of an incentive without complete deduction."[31]

As policymakers explored these private health insurance proposals, Allanson Willcox explains, "and the extent of governmental regulation that they would require became apparent, they lost their appeal even to people who wanted a voluntary approach."[32] Regulation of the insurance industry had traditionally been the states' responsibility, and any attempt at coordinating a universal strategy of insurance regulation among all the disparate states would have been unprecedented, extremely difficult, and unattractive.[33] What politicians sought was something simple and proven.

Eventually, Social Security began to emerge as a logical remedy for solving private health insurance's stubborn problems. The increasing returns that the 1950 amendments fostered made the program bigger, more generous, and extremely popular. After repeated failures to promote a sufficient expansion of private insurance, Pond explained, even Republicans in Congress began to look to Social Security as an alternative remedy due to its simplicity:

> Social Security is understood by every old person in the United States. They either get it or they don't get it. Most of them get it. Most of them rely on it to pay for most of their groceries and their rent and their clothing and their entertainment and the like. This is easy for them to understand. It's a regular system. They pay for it and they expect it as their right and due. But anything that is reasonably complicated—and I must confess that the Republican [Eisenhower] alternative was complicated—is very hard to describe.[34]

To its advantage, Social Security was not complicated. Its widespread familiarity and popularity with both government leaders and the public encouraged policy entrepreneurs to continue their incremental push for universal health insurance coverage.

Public Path: The Potential of Social Security's Expansion

The increasing returns that followed from Social Security's 1950 amendments contributed mightily to both the program's institutionalization and its capacity for expansion. What follows is an examination of how its increasing returns led to program expansion (including disability insurance) and why these events made Social Security ever more important for the future of universal public health insurance coverage.

Increasing Returns Protect and Nurture Social Security's OASI

Increasing returns associated with Social Security served to preclude any dramatic changes to the program during Eisenhower's administration. As the first Republican president since the introduction of Social Security, Eisenhower was not a social insurance advocate as his two predecessors had been. He did not share their public policy goals or embrace their core convictions. Yet Eisenhower's recommendations—together with the policy-making process that evolved from the constraints his Republican administration imposed—transformed Social Security into more than just a social welfare program. It became a formidably bipartisan political institution.

The minutes of Eisenhower's cabinet meetings devoted to the discussion of OASI reveal that the president's advisers considered the program to be "humane, forward, yet not New Dealish, founded on conservative principles of self-reliance."[35] Because Social Security was a "social mechanism for the preservation of individual dignity," they viewed it as a conservative institution that strengthened individualistic values.[36] An alternative plan championed by Social Security's archenemy (Republican Congressman Carl Curtis)—entitled the "Chamber of Commerce" program—called for a monthly stipend to be given to every retiree. But Eisenhower's cabinet derided the Chamber of Commerce plan as "bad math" and a "numbers racket . . . that we would always lose."[37]

Table 4.3
Percentage Increases in Prices and OASI Benefits, 1950-59

Date Of Change	Increase in OASI Benefit		Increase in Consumer Price Index	
	Each Amendment	Since January 1940	Each Amendment	Since January 1940
1950	81.3%	81.3%	75.5%	75.5%
1952	14.1	106.9	9.3	91.8
1954	13.3	134.3	0.5	92.8
1956*	—	—	—	—
1958	7.7	152.4	7.9	108.0

Source: Adapted and modified from Martha Derthick, *Policymaking for Social Security*
(Washington, D.C.: The Brookings Institution, 1970), table 13.1, 276.
* passage of disability insurance in this year

Not only did Eisenhower become supportive of Social Security, he even came to boast of his expansion of the program in campaign speeches. Early in 1954, he recommended, and Congress passed, a number of changes to OASI, including: (1) a 13 percent increase in monthly benefits; (2) a liberalized retirement-earnings provision; (3) the extension of the program to cover 10.5 million additional workers; (4) an increase in the level of taxable earnings from $3,600 to $4,200; and (5) a rise in the payroll tax rate to 2 percent. The last three recommendations significantly increased the amount of money in the program's trust fund. This surge in tax revenues made it easier for Congress to extend bigger benefits to many retirees who became newly covered, most of whom had never made any significant payroll contributions to the program.[38] The margin of victory for Eisenhower's recommendations in Congress was 356-8 in the House, and by unanimous voice vote in the Senate.[39]

Table 4.4
OASDI's Growing Generosity and Expanding Coverage, 1950-70

Year	Recipient/ Beneficiaries	Percentage of the population 65 and over	Average Monthly Benefit	Contributors/ Taxpayers	Taxpayers per Beneficiary
1950	3,477,000	16	$43.86	48,283,000	13.9
1955	7,961,000	—	61.90	65,203,000	8.2
1960	14,157,000	60	74.04	75,530,000	5.1
1965	19,128,000	—	83.92	80,681,000	4.2
1970	24,564,000	82	118.10	92,700,000	3.9

Source: Adapted from Robert Myers, *Social Security* (Bryn Mawr, Pa.: McCahan Foundation, 1975), tables 10.26, 10.27, 386-87.

Before Eisenhower left office, Congress expanded Social Security, either through OASI benefits or program additions such as disability insurance, in five straight election years: 1950, 1952, 1954, 1956, and 1958 (table 4.3). Part of elected leaders' motivation was to keep the program's benefits commensurate with inflation. But the fact that these increases came in election years and regularly exceeded the rise in prices suggests a more strategic mode of behavior by members of Congress with reelection in mind.

Collective bargaining, which propelled private health insurance, also played a big part in OASI's growth. New agreements between employers and unions in the 1950s required employers to provide pensions that would make up the difference between OASI and some fixed amount. Consequently, corporations and small businesses designed their retirement programs to mesh with OASI eligibility criteria. The value of an employee's pension would be pegged to the anticipated worth of his or her monthly OASI check. It is little wonder then that companies such as Ford were some of the leading voices in the 1950s calling for increased OASI benefits, to relieve them of the major responsibility for making sure retirees' pensions were adequate.[40] Between 1950 and 1970, the number of OASI beneficiaries jumped over 677 percent; average monthly benefits more than doubled from $43.86 to $118.10; wage-earning contributors to the program rose from 48 to 93 million; and increases in OASI benefits exceeded inflation by 40 percent (table 4.4).[41]

With these increases in benefits and beneficiaries, Social Security became immensely popular with the public, the Eisenhower administration, and virtually every senator and representative. The program's perceived success stemmed from its actuarial soundness (at least on paper) and its massive cash distribution. As welfare-state historian Edward Berkowitz points out, in the 1950s and 1960s:

Politicians celebrated Social Security as a characteristically American institution, a marvelous mix of pluralism and pragmatism, a sure winner in Congress because of the way it transferred money to the elderly even as policymakers lauded the way it reinforced the American tradition of self-reliance.

Those decades provided ideal conditions in which to nurture a social insurance program. Wages were rising, and as they rose, more money flowed into the Social Security trust funds. Unemployment remained at low levels. . . . Fertility rates continued at high levels, insuring a high worker to beneficiary ratio far into the future as more babies grew up and had babies of their own. . . . Since the trust funds were chock full of money, it did not seem a disgraceful matter to vote a Social Security benefit increase, and if the increase came in an election year, well, that was simply a fortunate happenstance.[42]

Disability Insurance: First Step Toward Health Insurance

Social Security's popularity became a strategic asset for those pursuing universal coverage. Tired of continually losing to organized medicine represented by the AMA, social insurance enthusiasts changed their strategy in the early 1950s to seek more modest goals. Specifically, Oscar Ewing, President Truman's federal security administrator, decided in 1950 to pursue a narrower, incrementally targeted health insurance program.[43] According to Ewing, the Wagner-Murray-Dingell Bills, which proposed almost cradle-to-grave protection by the government for all individuals, were politically impractical.[44]

To add health insurance coverage to Social Security, SSA administrators believed the first step was disability insurance.[45] "The major thrust during the early 1950s was not Medicare or health insurance," Arthur Hess, SSA program analyst and later director of disability insurance, pointed out. "The major program thrust, from the point of view of labor and the Democratic administration or the Democrats in Congress and some of the old Social Security planners from way back, was to get disability insurance."[46]

Health insurance aside, achieving a disability insurance program required incremental steps of its own. The first one came in 1954, when SSA administrators persuaded Congress that it was both unnecessary and unfair for workers to lose much of their OASI benefits because of a permanent disability.[47] Congress responded by passing what became known as a "disability freeze." Introduced in 1954, it prevented workers from losing their OASI benefits due to a career-ending illness before the age of sixty-five.[48] "The freeze preserved a disabled worker's rights to social security at age sixty-five," explains Berkowitz. "Under its terms, persons who became disabled had their benefit records 'frozen.'"[49]

The freeze for OASI benefits provided the key step to an actual program of disability insurance. The AMA strongly opposed it, because it sensed that a disability program was a first step toward national health insurance. But Social Security's popularity made it hard for many in Congress to resist using the program to help workers who were permanently disabled. In due course, the disability freeze led Congress to take another step: the passing of a full-fledged disability program in 1956.[50] It was a major victory for SSA executives and leaders of organized labor. Incrementalism continued two years later in 1958, when Congress made the dependents of disability beneficiaries eligible for benefits. And in 1960, it removed the requirement that recipients be at least fifty years old.[51]

SSA administrators' victory in passing disability insurance represented the first time the AMA lost a major public-policy dispute. It showed advocates of social insurance that they could defeat organized medicine if they proposed a program conservative enough to neutralize doctors' leading objections.[52] Disability insurance also revealed that while the AMA might dominate policy-making in the private sector, it had difficulty opposing a minor program addition to Social Security, intended to relieve the suffering of a uniquely vulnerable group of older individuals.

Passing disability insurance required political compromise and pragmatism, which SSA administrators had honed to exquisite levels. Learning from the experience of disability insurance, Edwin Witte—one of Social Security's original architects—made the following argument in 1958 for the next incremental step, health insurance:

> I recognize that compulsory health insurance cannot be established at this time over the opposition of the AMA and our strong American preference for voluntary action. It seems more likely that we will continue to increase tax-supported public medical care rather than consider the taboo, compulsory health insurance. The wisest course may be not to aim for a complete national system of health insurance, but to supplement voluntary health insurance by a government program of hospital insurance for the old-age beneficiaries.[53]

Disability insurance not only was a triumph for incrementalism, as Martha Derthick asserts, it was a "necessary prelude" to Medicare.[55]

Conclusion

Following 1950, Social Security experienced a period of tremendous growth due to increasing returns that made it more and more attractive. This growth was largely financed by the program's "level earnings assumption," in which administrators made actuarial predictions based on the (implausible) assumption that wages would remain constant. Instead, when wages rose every year—as economists and politicians knew they would—the "unexpected surplus" provided Congress easy money to pay for increased benefits.[55] This annual event, along with the 1950 amendments, constituted in effect a conscious, collective decision on the part of Congress to champion OASI by greatly increasing both the size of the program's benefits and the number of its beneficiaries. The result is that OASI became further institutionalized as the dominant program for retirement pensions.

Similarly, the failure of Truman's ambitious national health proposal and the subsequent rise of collective bargaining led to a massive increase in private coverage. Blue Cross/Blue Shield and corporate health insurance became the primary means by which people protected themselves against the cost of illness. In both areas, individuals and organizations adjusted their behavior to the new incentives that increasing returns produced. Over time these returns served to cement the dominant roles of private health insurance and Social Security.

Perhaps most important, though, the meteoric rise of health insurance fostered a number of problems for groups that remained excluded—the poor, disabled, unemployed, and retirees. When attempts to remedy these problems with private solutions failed, Social Security began to emerge as the alternative solution. This development launched policymakers' incremental drive for a public health insurance path, starting with disability insurance. Their passage of disability insurance in 1956 demonstrated that effective use of policy learning could overcome the AMA's interest group opposition.[56] Incrementally building on Social Security's success and popularity became the means by which policymakers could pass a public health insurance scheme.

Notes

1. Robert Myers, *Social Security* (Bryn Mawr, Pa.: McCahan Foundation, 1975), 386-87, tables 10.26, 10.27.

2. Agnes Brewster, "Voluntary Health Insurance and Medical Care Expenditures," *Social Security Bulletin* 21, no. 12 (December 1958): 13, table 6. See also, Health Insurance Association of America, *Source Book of Health Insurance Data* (Washington, D.C.: Health Insurance Association of America, 1991), 24.

3. Howard Jacob Karger and David Stoesz, *American Social Welfare Policy: A Pluralist Approach* (New York: Longman, 1998), 210: "The term collective bargaining refers to the face-to-face interaction between unionized employees and management for the purposes of negotiating a group contract."

4. Paul Pierson, "When Effect Becomes Cause," *World Politics* 45 (July 1993): 608. See also, Paul Romer, "Increasing Returns and Long-Run Growth," *Journal of Political Economy* 94 (1986): 1002-37.

5. Paul Pierson, "Increasing Returns, Path Dependence, and the Study of Politics," Program for the Study of Germany and Europe, Working Paper Series 7.7 (Center for European Studies, Harvard University, September 1, 1997), 19.

6. Pierson, "Increasing Returns, Path Dependence, and the Study of Politics," Working Paper Series 7.7, 8.

7. Pierson, "When Effect Becomes Cause," 609. See also, Brian Arthur, *Increasing Returns and Path Dependence in the Economy* (Ann Arbor: University of Michigan Press, 1994); Douglass C. North, *Institutions, Institutional Change, and Economic Performance* (New York: Cambridge University Press, 1990); Stephen Krasner, "Sovereignty: An Institutional Perspective," *Comparative Political Studies* 21 (April 1988): 66-94; and John Ikenberry, "History's Heavy Hand: Institutions and the Politics of the

State," paper presented at the Conference on "New Institutionalism," University of Maryland (October 14-15, 1994).

8. For more on this subject, see Arthur F. McClure, *The Truman Administration and the Problems of Postwar Labor, 1945-1948* (Rutherford, N.J.: Fairleigh Dickinson Press, 1969).

9. See Michael K. Brown, "Bargaining for Social Rights: Unions and the Reemergence of Welfare Capitalism," *Political Science Quarterly* 112, no. 4 (Winter 1997): 645-75.

10. Interview with Alanson Willcox, Oral History Collection, Columbia University (1967), 53. (Hereafter Willcox, OHC.)

11. Interview with James Brindle and Martin Cohen, Oral History Collection, Columbia University (1967), 4-6. (Hereafter Brindle and Cohen, OHC.) For more on the impressive growth in private health insurance programs through collective bargaining, see Frank R. Dobbin, "The Origins of Private Social Insurance: Public Policy and Fringe Benefits in America, 1920-1950," *American Journal of Sociology* 97, no. 5 (March 1992): 1416-50.

12. See *Inland Steel Company v. United Steel Workers of America* (CIO), 77 NLRB 4 (1948); and the Supreme Court's reaffirmation of *Inland Co. v. NLRB*, U.S. Court of Appeals, 7th Circuit (September 23, 1948). See also, Beth Stevens, "Blurring the Boundaries: How the Federal Government Has Influenced Welfare Benefits in the Private Sector," in *The Politics of Social Policy in the United States*, ed. M. Weir, A. Orloff, and T. Skocpol (Princeton, N.J.: Princeton University Press, 1988), 140-41: "The conflict over collective bargaining with regard to employee benefits came to a head in 1948 in a landmark case that was decided by the National Labor Relations Board (NLRB). The steelworkers had sought to bargain with the Inland Steel Company over its policy of compulsory retirement. The company refused to bargain, arguing that the policy was contained in a provision of its pension plan and therefore not subject to collective bargaining. In April 1948, the NLRB ruled against Inland Steel, stating that the Taft-Hartley Act required employers to bargain over pensions. Pensions, it held, came within the meaning of the term 'conditions of employment' that the legislation had identified as an appropriate topic for bargaining. Two months later, in the *W. W. Cross* case, the board extended its ruling to group insurance. In early 1949 it ruled that General Motors could not institute a group insurance plan without first consulting with the union."

13. See Hugh H. Macaulay Jr., *Fringe Benefits and Their Federal Tax Treatment* (New York: Columbia University Press, 1959), 8-15.

14. Paul Starr, *The Social Transformation of American Medicine* (New York: Basic Books, 1982), 313. See also, H. M. Douty, "Post-war Wage Bargaining in the United States," in *Labor and Trade Unionism*, ed. Walter Galenson and Seymour Martin Lipset (New York: Wiley, 1960), 192-202.

15. Macaulay, *Fringe Benefits and Their Federal Tax Treatment*, 13: "Although cash wages are the traditional weapon used in this battle [the competition among employers for workers], fringe benefits have become more important as a supplementary artillery piece. . . . [T]hese benefits not only attract new workers to the firm but they also help the firm to hold on to its workers and to improve the productivity of these workers."

16. Thomas A. Kochan, Harry C. Katz, and Robert B. McKersie, *The Transformation of American Industrial Relations* (Ithaca, N.Y.: ILR Press, 1994), 31-35.

17. Kochan, Katz, and McKersie, *The Transformation of American Industrial Relations*, 33: "This agreement, which lasted for two years, instituted cost-of-living and annual improvement-factor wage increases; included grievance and arbitration procedures;

provided an array of fringe benefits, including pension, health, and insurance benefits; and was followed in 1950 by a five-year agreement that included these clauses."

18. Kochan, Katz, and McKersie, *The Transformation of American Industrial Relations*, 30, 35.

19. Joseph W. Garbarino, *Health Plans and Collective Bargaining* (Berkeley: University of California Press, 1960), 279-84. See also, Raymond Munts, *Bargaining for Health: Labor Unions, Health Insurance, and Medical Care* (Madison, Wis.: University of Wisconsin Press, 1960).

20. Brewster, "Voluntary Health Insurance and Medical Care Expenditures," 13, table 6. See also, A. Somers and H. Somers, *Health and Health Care: Policies in Perspective* (Germantown, Md.: Aspen Systems Corporation, 1977), 109; U.S. Chamber of Commerce, *Fringe Benefits, 1953* (Washington, D.C.: GPO, 1954); and National Industrial Conference Board, *Computing the Cost of Fringe Benefits* (Studies in Personnel Policy, no. 128), New York, 1952.

21. Brewster, "Voluntary Health Insurance and Medicare Care Expenditures," 13. See also, Health Insurance Association of America, *Source Book of Health Insurance Data* (Washington, D.C.: Health Insurance Association of America, 1991), 24.

22. Marie Gottschalk, *The Shadow Welfare State: Labor, Business, and the Politics of Health Care in the United States* (Ithaca, N.Y.: Cornell University Press, 2000), 48.

23. Gottschalk, *The Shadow Welfare State*, 47-48.

24. The following was a popular joke with numerous variations: "I have health insurance. If a giraffe bites me on the shoulder, I get $18, provided I'm pregnant at the time." By Phil Leeds in Richard Carter's *The Doctor Business* (New York: Doubleday, 1958), 96.

25. Odin Anderson, *Blue Cross since 1929* (Cambridge: Ballinger Publishing Company, 1975), 69-80. Experience rating refers to the practice of charging customers different premiums according to the risk they pose. For example, a young man in his mid-twenties would pay much less for health insurance than an old man in his mid-eighties, because the likelihood of the older man needing medical care would be significantly greater.

26. Interview with Katherine Ellickson, Oral History Collection, Columbia University (1969), 86.

27. Interview with Allen Pond, Oral History Collection, Columbia University (1966), 11. (Hereafter Pond, OHC.)

28. Stevens, "Blurring the Boundaries," 147.

29. Pond, OHC, 2.

30. Pond, OHC, 2-3: "The reinsurance idea had attractiveness in its early stages primarily because it could be designed to help spread the risk of covering poor risks. At that time insurance companies were loath to provide coverage for people who weren't in first-rate physical condition. They were quite reluctant. They'd had no experience at it really. They were quite reluctant to cover the aged or to cover people with disabilities. And the concept of the reinsurance plan was to try to make it possible for the government to set up a system that would protect the insurance companies and Blue Cross-Blue Shield plans against the losses resulting from their experimentation in new forms of coverage or in extended coverage."

31. Pond, OHC, 24-25.

32. Willcox, OHC, 54.

33. Pond, OHC, 26.

34. Pond, OHC, 66-67.

35. Folder "C-8 (4), November 20, 1953," White House Office, Office of the Staff Secretary, Cabinet Series, Box 1, Dwight D. Eisenhower Library, Abilene, Kans.; as cited in Mark H. Leff, "Historical Perspectives on Old-Age Insurance: The State of the Art on the Art of the State," in *Social Security after Fifty: Successes and Failures*, ed. Edward D. Berkowitz (New York: Greenwood Press, 1987), 33.

36. Andrew Achenbaum, *Social Security: Visions and Revisions* (Cambridge: Cambridge University Press, 1986), 48.

37. Folders "C-9 (3), December 15, 1993," 78-79 and "C-8 (4), November 20, 1953," 56, both in Box 1, White House Office, Office of the Staff Secretary, Cabinet Series, Eisenhower Library, Abilene, Kans.; as cited in Leff, "Historical Perspectives on Old-Age Insurance," 33.

38. Martha Derthick, *Policymaking for Social Security* (Washington, D.C.: The Brookings Institution, 1970), 6, n9: "An extreme individual example is Ida Fuller of Brattleboro, Vermont, who was in the program's first group of beneficiaries. She began getting social security checks on January 31, 1940. Miss Fuller had paid $22 in taxes before her retirement. When she died in a nursing home thirty-five years later at the age of one hundred, she had received more than $20,000 in benefits."

39. Gary W. Reichard's, *The Reaffirmation of Republicanism: Eisenhower and the Eighty-Third Congress* (Knoxville: University of Tennessee Press, 1975).

40. William Graebner, *A History of Retirement* (New Haven, Conn.: Yale University Press, 1970), ch. 8; Achenbaum, *Social Security: Visions and Revisions*, 46-47.

41. As measured by the Consumer Price Index: *Future Directions in Social Security*, Hearings before the Senate Special Committee on Aging, 93rd Congress, 1st session (Washington, D.C.: GPO, 1973), part 1, 84.

42. Edward D. Berkowitz, *America's Welfare State from Roosevelt to Reagan* (Baltimore: Johns Hopkins University Press, 1991), 66-67.

43. Willcox, OHC, 47.

44. Willcox, OHC, 47.

45. Philip Booth, *Social Security in America* (Ann Arbor: University of Michigan Press, 1973), 36.

46. Interview with Arthur Hess, Oral History Collection, Columbia University (1968), 20.

47. J. Douglas Brown, *An American Philosophy of Social Insurance: Evolution and Issues* (Princeton, N.J.: Princeton University Press, 1972), 156-57.

48. See Jerry L. Mashaw, "Disability Insurance in an Age of Retrenchment: The Politics of Implementing Rights," in *Social Security: Beyond the Rhetoric of Crisis*, ed. Theodore R. Marmor and Jerry K. Mashaw (Princeton, N.J.: Princeton University Press, 1988), 155.

49. Edward Berkowitz, *Disabled Policy: America's Programs for the Handicapped* (Cambridge: Cambridge University Press, 1987), 70: "If they qualified for benefits when their records were frozen, they received them when they reached retirement age, even though they had been out of the labor force and paying nothing into the social security trust fund."

50. Berkowitz, *American's Welfare State from Roosevelt to Reagan*, 165.

51. See W. L. Mitchell, "Social Security Legislation in the 86th Congress," *Social Security Bulletin* (November 1960): 3-29; and Brown, *An American Philosophy of Social Insurance*, 157.

52. Mashaw, "Disability Insurance in an Age of Retrenchment," 155: "Indeed, although the AMA fought [the 'disability freeze'], the provision was very difficult to op-

pose: a similar freeze was common in private health insurance, the proposal seemed eminently fair, and it cost very little."

53. Edwin E. Witte, "Excerpts from Address at the Meeting of the Catholic Economic Association at Chicago, December 28, 1958," *Review of Social Economy* 17 (March 1959): 31-32.

54. Derthick, *Policymaking for Social Security*, 319: "Much in the contest over disability insurance anticipated the later struggle over Medicare and helped to prepare program executives for it. There was the same process of cutting and trimming in an effort to mollify opposition and make the change seem a modest addition to old age insurance rather than a big new departure. There was the same responsive, pragmatic accommodation to intermediary organizations that would have a big role in administration. . . . There was the same decision in Congress to enact first the public assistance alternative— a categorical grant-in-aid program for the disabled in 1950, and a program of medical assistance for the aged in 1960.

More than a political trial run for Medicare, the passage of disability insurance was a necessary prelude. The drive for health insurance would not be resumed until disability coverage was safely out of the way, but once it was out of the way, program executives did not lose a moment."

55. Derthick, *Policymaking for Social Security*, 350-55, 385-86.

56. Essentially, social insurance advocates could employ one form of policy feedback (policy learning) to neutralize the hindering effects of another (interest group activity).

CHAPTER FIVE

Symbiotic Attachment

"Health Insurance through Social Security"
(early 1960s through early 1970s)

> *In 1935 when the man that both of us loved so much, Franklin Delano Roosevelt, signed the Social Security Act, he said it was, and I quote him, "a cornerstone in a structure which is being built but . . . is by no means complete." Well, perhaps no single act in his entire administration really did more to win him the illustrious place in history that he has, as did the laying of that cornerstone. Those who share this day will . . . be remembered for making the most important addition to that structure. . . . We marvel not simply at the passage of this bill, but what we marvel at is that it took so many years for it to pass.*
>
> **—President Lyndon B. Johnson**
> with former President Harry S Truman
> Signing of Medicare (July 30, 1965)

The decade between the early 1960s and early 1970s represents policymakers' most successful period for incrementally expanding social insurance.[1] Specifically, the seven years from 1965 to 1972 constitute Social Security's "glory days." As a strategy, incrementalism came by way of policy learning, which provided social insurance advocates a way for finally overcoming the interest group opposition of organized medicine (AMA).[2] The key to greatly improving the political prospects of a program such as Medicare, policymakers learned, was to attach it to Social Security.

In pursuing incrementalism, political actors' critical source of policy learning came from the impact of previously adopted policies.[3] Generally, how policymakers respond to any social need is largely determined by how they have successfully and unsuccessfully addressed similar issues in the past.[4] Policymakers in the early 1960s learned from their previous mistakes and, in turn, crafted more workable proposals that capitalized on Social Security's popularity.

61

For many of the program's founding architects, the momentous passage of Medicare in 1965 partially fulfilled their original goal of including health insurance as part of Social Security. And they hoped that Medicare might propel the strategy of incrementalism to the point of reaching universal coverage.

An analysis of both Medicare's passage and policymakers' subsequent success in enlarging Social Security's OASDI benefits between 1966 and 1972 is intended to answer a number of specific questions. Why were policymakers finally successful in passing Medicare in contrast to many failed attempts between 1935 and 1964? Was Medicare the product of a relentless incrementalism that finally pushed over the goal line? Or was it, as Lawrence Brown argues, "an anomalous consequence of political convergences and coalitions so rare that they dominate U.S. politics for perhaps ten years in a century, and are neither directly producible nor predictable?"[5] Last, what were the implications of Medicare and OASDI's huge benefit increases for the goal of universal coverage?

The Road to Medicare: Incrementalism in Earnest

The Forand Bill, first introduced in Congress in 1957, marked the formal (albeit modest) beginning of social insurance advocates' incremental crusade for Medicare.[6] One year after the successful passage of disability insurance, the Forand Bill was the first-ever plan intended to provide health insurance for the elderly. Named after Congressman Aime Forand (D-R.I.), the bill received the endorsement only of organized labor. No other interest group of any significance supported the plan. Republicans in Congress vehemently opposed it. Allen Pond, an Eisenhower appointee at the Department of Health, Education, and Welfare (HEW), observed that Eisenhower was absolutely committed to private, voluntary alternatives.[7] "This is going to be a ten-year fight," Congressman Forand privately told friends. "I know just what we're going to be up against. It's going to be a ten-year fight."[8] The Forand Bill died twice, once in 1957 and again in a similar incarnation in 1959.[9] But by 1960 congressmen were receiving more mail on health care and the Forand proposal than any other legislative issue.[10]

Unable to advance their own social insurance plan, advocates such as Wilbur Cohen learned they could capitalize on the flaws and shortcomings of private insurance—which were becoming increasingly acute for many families—to educate and influence members of Congress. In particular, the term "three-generation family" became common. It signified how a growing number of middle-aged couples found themselves simultaneously providing for their children's education and their parents' medical bills.[11] Medicare advocates used the term to increase awareness among the public and Congress of the problem. "I think experience has been that a long period of preparation is usually necessary before you can get legislation through and, therefore, you don't wait until the situation is entirely ripe," observed Katherine Ellickson. "You have to educate people and they have to talk to their Congressman . . . and you have to get it in the papers and so on."[12] While policymakers learned from their mistakes, the Forand Bill raised the issue of health insurance for the elderly to a position that demanded action. Congress finally responded, but it began with a welfare proposal called Kerr-Mills.

Waiting with Welfare: From Kerr-Mills to Medicare

Patience was a critical element in the incremental pursuit of Medicare. Generally, policymakers often had to wait for years while Congress first tried to solve a policy problem with a welfare program. Frequently, events vindicated their patience when the welfare scheme would give way to a social insurance alternative. In effect, policymakers would replace introductory "starter" plans with more mature and improved programs. For example, old age insurance operated in the shadow of old age assistance until after 1950, when it switched and became the dominant program. Disability insurance, which Congress passed in 1956 as an addition to Social Security, replaced a disability welfare program begun in 1950. In both instances, only after a welfare program failed did Congress finally turn to social insurance. Over time, Elizabeth Wickenden argues, social insurance became more attractive than welfare for financial and political reasons.[13]

Hoping that it could alleviate the need for a social insurance program such as the one proposed in the Forand Bill, Congress passed a welfare alternative in 1960 called Kerr-Mills. Designed largely by Wilbur Cohen and named after its sponsors, Congressman Wilbur Mills (chairman of the House Ways and Means Committee) and Senator Robert Kerr (chairman of the Senate Finance Committee), Kerr-Mills extended federal support to individual states for taking care of the health needs of impoverished elderly persons.[14] Robert Myers, Social Security's chief actuary from 1938 to 1970 and the authority throughout his tenure on the financial viability of program adjustment, recalls the origins of Kerr-Mills:

> [I]t came about largely because Mr. Mills and Senator Kerr didn't want the social insurance approach. Their fear was that this would burgeon on out and destroy a lot of private insurance and eventually develop into national health insurance or even socialized medicine.[15]

For a social insurance program such as Medicare to pass, the welfare alternative of Kerr-Mills first had to fail. Conveniently, it began to do so shortly after its passage. According to Elliot Richardson (President Eisenhower's assistant secretary for legislation and secretary of HEW under Nixon), by 1963 only four states provided the full range of care for which Kerr-Mills allowed. Furthermore, the five large industrial states—California, New York, Massachusetts, Michigan, and Pennsylvania—were receiving upwards of 90 percent of all federal matching funds, while their elderly populations represented just 33 percent of the total country's population over the age of sixty-five.[16] Disillusioned by his own program as early as 1962, Mills disliked having his name attached to something that created so much dissatisfaction and frustration.[17]

Although the Kerr-Mills program ultimately failed, it provided an important encouragement to SSA leaders, organized labor, and liberal congressmen. It represented Congress's first programmatic response to the issue of health insurance for retirees, admitting that something had to be done. Moreover, Kerr-Mills served to greatly increase the public's familiarity with and tolerance for a future program such as Medicare. This made it a critical stepping-stone toward adding some measure of health insurance coverage to Social Security. The primary obstacles Medicare supporters would have to overcome were organized medicine and Wilbur Mills.

Medicare's Two Main Hurdles: The AMA and Wilbur Mills

As expected, organized medicine became Medicare's primary foe. Given the number of health insurance proposals it had defeated, dating back as far as individual state initiatives in the 1920s, its political strength was intimidating. Perhaps organized medicine's most formidable advantage came in the person of Mills, whose steadfast personal commitment to the AMA greatly disadvantaged Medicare's prospects. Only a handful of individuals knew of Mills's commitment at the time, and it has still not become widely known. But as Blue Carstenson, head of the National Council of Senior Citizens (NCSC) at the time, later told an interviewer:

> One of the reasons I knew that it was going to be difficult for Wilbur Mills to buy this [Medicare] is that Mills was originally backed by a small group of doctors in Arkansas when he ran against the incumbent when he originally got his first seat. He never forgot that, that he originally owed his seat to a group of doctors who financed his campaign in Arkansas. So the chances of him working out something this way didn't seem to be at all tenable to us.[18]

Mills's devotion to the AMA, along with his conservative approach to expanding Social Security, made incrementalism an exceedingly slow and frustrating process. "I never did think they had a chance until 1964," said the SSA's chief actuary, Robert Myers: "Most of the people in the Social Security Administration always thought that they were going to persuade Mr. Mills, which was the vote they needed in essence." Yet, Myers added, "It seemed to me that he was just leading them on and on, asking them more questions, putting up more hurdles for them to jump."[19] Not until after Lyndon Johnson's victory in 1964 did the political balance of Ways and Means change. Mills then altered his views, because had he not he would have lost control of his committee.[20]

The previous incremental victory of disability insurance chipped away at the AMA's influence. Congressmen became less intimidated by the organization. Their experience with disability insurance showed not only that the AMA's predictions sometimes were inaccurate, but also that its opposition could be inconsistent. The SSA's deputy commissioner by 1970, Arthur Hess, recalls how organized medicine lost its ability to frighten legislators into supporting its positions:

I think that over time Congressmen either got completely fed up with the AMA representation or came to the conclusion that not only was it not the kiss of death, but a lot of the things that were predicted (you know, there were such dire predictions about what would happen if disability insurance was enacted) were imaginary. What happened with disability insurance then helped to demonstrate that none of these dire predictions came to pass, nobody was regimented, nobody was socialized, and doctors didn't lose their patients.

Q: And doctors also didn't punish the people who had voted for disability?

That's right. . . . I think it demonstrated to Congressmen and others that there was by no means this unity of point of view in the medical profession; that even though the spokesmen of organized medicine predicted doom, the facts were that many individual physicians were perfectly satisfied with the way things were going.[21]

In desperation, the AMA made a critical decision that later handicapped the organization in its battle against Medicare. Aware of its declining influence, organized medicine decided to ditch its opposition to government involvement in health insurance. In 1960, it came out in support of the Kerr-Mills Bill after having previously opposed the plan.[22] In supporting Kerr-Mills, though, organized medicine admitted that something had to be done on behalf of the elderly. After Kerr-Mills failed both administratively and politically, consideration of Medicare started from a more advanced position. Doing nothing was no longer an option after 1960, as it had been in all previous health insurance debates. Policymakers possessed little doubt that a new policy would eventually replace Kerr-Mills, but its final structure remained unknown.

Organized Labor

Labor played the largest role of any interest group in pushing the incremental strategy on behalf of Medicare. According to Lee Bamberger and Leonard Lesser, policy leaders for organized labor, the "AFL-CIO became a sort of headquarters offering at least logistical support—that is, desks and mimeograph machines—for the people who were trying to get something done about health insurance for the aged. I can remember the library in the IUD [Industrial Union Department] when we were assembling, cutting and pasting a bill."[23] When the leadership of Medicare's campaign shifted to the Kennedy administration starting in 1961, the organized labor-SSA relationship remained critical in keeping Medicare on the policy agenda. James Brindle, a leader of the United Auto Workers at the time, described the relationship: "It's interesting the way the policy stuff used to get done. We worked very closely with the Social Security people. . . . We backed the SSA on this stuff and used to work with them and help develop it."[24] Because unions had already secured generous health insurance benefits for their workers through collective bargaining agreements with employers (see chapter 4), they no longer had any driving interest in national health insurance.

Instead, they wanted a targeted, scaled-down addition to Social Security that would not threaten their private arrangements. Medicare offered just such a convenient scheme. Not only would it relieve middle-aged workers from having to pay their parents' medical bills, but later it would also act as a suitable addendum to their own health insurance needs when they retired.

Learning from its previous failures in battling the AMA, labor sought an ally to avoid a solitary confrontation with organized medicine—a fight that labor firmly believed it would lose. Nelson Cruikshank, AFL-CIO's chief policy strategist, explains the rationale for incorporating other interest groups, namely retirees, on its behalf:

> [Here is] the argument—Look, labor can't do this alone. It's got to be more than a labor cause. The old people are interested in this, but they're inarticulate, they have no way of channeling their influence to Congress, they don't know how to be effective with Congress. They've got to have a paper, a bulletin, a little staff of field people and people that can talk their own language, appeal to their own interests, get them to take part in political action and legislative action. And the labor movement can't do this. . . . You need a broader base and this is the way to get it.[25]

The outcome of labor's efforts to broaden political support was creation in 1960 of the National Council of Senior Citizens, which began its operation in the national offices of the United Steelworkers of America.[26] The relationship between labor and retirees was not always harmonious. "There were days when we would say, 'We could do our work a whole lot better if there were no senior citizens' organizations,'" remembered the AFL-CIO's Lee Bamberger.[27] Her colleague, Leonard Lesser, admitted that labor had another major concern—it "did not want to start another Townsend movement."[28]

But despite labor's fears about its political involvement with senior citizens, the elderly proved to be of enormous strategic help in disseminating effective propaganda. Between 1950 and 1963, the number of senior citizens grew from approximately 12 million to 17.5 million, 10 percent of the overall population. Meanwhile, the costs of hospital care continued to rise 6.7 percent a year, far in excess of the annual increase in the cost of living. Consequently, private health insurers continually increased their insurance premiums. So by 1964, only one in four senior citizens had complete health insurance coverage.[29] The NCSC's Blue Carstenson illustrates how supporters of Medicare learned to capitalize on the elderly's plight:

> You would hit a real good story when you'd talk with a reporter and he would have already had to shell out money for his mother's hospitalization or his aunt's hospitalization or the mother was living with them and they were afraid any day she was going to get a heart attack and they'd have to come up with the money because she was canceled out of Blue Cross. This was where we really got our biggest press play, if you could latch onto some reporter with a problem. So you'd play this when you were talking to the press. You'd get into

what this meant to individuals and talk about their own grandparents. . . . Before you knew it, they were talking. Pretty soon they were enthusiastic for the bill, too, and away you'd go.[30]

Efforts by organized labor and social insurance enthusiasts—such as the one recalled by Blue Carstenson—to publicize the elderly's plight began to show dividends. Recognizing the elderly's peculiar vulnerability, public opinion in favor of Medicare grew during the 1964 presidential campaign and after Lyndon Johnson's victory.[31] In January 1965, the Gallup organization polled 1,564 Americans regarding health insurance, asking: "Congress has been considering a compulsory medical insurance program covering hospital and nursing home care for the elderly. This Medicare program would be financed out of increased Social Security taxes. In general, do you approve or disapprove of this program?" A resounding 63 percent of those queried said they approved of the program, compared with 28 percent who disapproved and 9 percent who said they did not know.

Benefits by Right versus the Means Test

The growing success of Medicare advocates' incrementalist strategy resulted in increased bipartisan support for the proposal. Medicare's image of "benefits by right" helps to explain why it (and Social Security for that matter) engendered strong support across the ideological spectrum. The program's designers incorporated a self-financing mechanism that conservatives liked, with relatively generous, universal benefits appreciated by liberals. Most of the public preferred Medicare's social insurance structure to welfare assistance, because Medicare did not involve a means test for someone to receive the program's benefits. The program's advantage was its emphasis on "human dignity."[32]

The public's dislike of means testing reflected another key element of Medicare. Its financing was successfully portrayed not only as progressive[33] but also as "class blind." In other words, a manual laborer would contribute less in Medicare payroll taxes—and the same monthly Part B premium—than a wealthy financier, but their benefits would be identical. As Arthur Hess, the SSA's commissioner in 1974, told an interviewer:

Of course, historically there are a lot of threads and relationships that you like to trace through, but it seems to me that the average Congressman who voted for Medicare or who became convinced that Medicare was necessary, and the average American who's for it or against it, hasn't got the slightest interest, recollection or philosophical disposition to think of this in terms at all of the kind of basic theories and issues and concerns that you get when you trace through the history of health insurance proposals. To me this was a very pragmatic response to a need which existed in the middle of this particular century. . . . [I]t got right down to the point where it was an issue of "right" versus the "means test," and I think the public had a pretty good idea on that one.[34]

Once health insurance for retirees ceased to be a theoretical problem (with the passage of Kerr-Mills in 1960), it became primarily a logistical one. This development suited SSA leaders and the pragmatic incrementalism they pursued. They improved Medicare's appeal by incorporating the services of private intermediaries in the program's technical operation. Instead of hospitals and doctors dealing directly with the federal government for reimbursement, they would interface with private entities such as corporate insurance carriers and Blue Cross/Blue Shield. These intermediaries, in turn, would then complete the transaction with the federal government.[35]

With private intermediaries, Medicare's final structure, Part A for hospital insurance and Part B for medical insurance or physicians' fees, closely mirrored the existing nonprofit structure of Blue Cross (hospital insurance) and Blue Shield (medical insurance). Adopting this private policy structure served to undercut the AMA's political opposition. "Now, the AMA could not deny the validity of the appropriateness of the approach of Blue Cross and Blue Shield," noted Cruikshank. "After all, Blue Shield was their baby; Blue Cross was the American Hospital Association, and while they had shifted positions since 1933, the AMA at this time was saying that Blue Cross/Blue Shield and private and commercial insurance were the correct approach."[36] The stage was set for Medicare's passage.

Medicare: The "Three-Layered-Cake"

Just as Franklin Roosevelt's victory in 1932 made Social Security possible, Lyndon Johnson's in 1964 did the same for Medicare. According to Theodore Marmor, "The electoral outcome of 1964 guaranteed the passage of legislation on medical care for the aged."[37] President Johnson won by the largest plurality in history. In addition, House Democrats gained thirty-eight seats, resulting in a 295-140 majority over Republicans, and Senate Democrats increased their daunting majority by two seats to 68-32.

Overwhelmed by the enormity of Johnson's and the Democrats' victory, Wilbur Mills finally succumbed: "I can support a payroll tax for financing health benefits just as I have supported a payroll tax for cash benefits."[39] Mills later confided to an interviewer that Johnson's landslide election made Medicare's passage inevitable: "Johnson espoused it in his campaign, you know, and here was elected by a 2 to 1 vote, which was a pretty strong endorsement of it, I thought. I thought the time had come to pass it."[39] So massive was Johnson's landslide that it even translated into critical change to the Ways and Means Committee. According to Mills, "The House went two to one, so the committee was set up two-to-one. We had fewer Republicans and more Democrats; the only time we had a change."[40]

Republicans and organized medicine became desperate following Mills's capitulation and the Democrats' large numerical increase in Congress. The AMA responded first with a new strategy of introducing a voluntary, alternative private plan called "Eldercare." The program called for more comprehensive benefits for the elderly, including insurance for physicians' services.[41] Having lost out on the supply of clever phraseology, the Republicans rallied around yet another alternative called "Better-Care." It was more a diversionary tactic than a serious proposal. Better-Care—like the AMA's Eldercare—would have been voluntary, and financed from both the federal government's general revenues and monthly "premiums" paid by participating senior citizens.[42]

The Republicans' Better-Care proposal provided Chairman Mills with a unique opportunity for reconciliation. He combined Johnson's Medicare proposal for hospital insurance with Republicans' Better-Care plan for physician's services into a "three-layered cake" that included Medicaid,[43] a Kerr-Mills (means-tested) plan for the poor. The Johnson administration's plan became Medicare Part A (hospital insurance), and the Republicans' Better-Care plan, scaled down, became Medicare Part B (physicians' services). Part A would be financed by a small expansion of Social Security's payroll tax to be diverted into a separate trust fund. Part B would be jointly financed by general revenues and the monthly premiums of participating senior citizens.

Mills's unusual three-layered cake had a hidden logic to it. He recognized that social insurance advocates' strategic use of incrementalism had triumphed for the purposes of hospital insurance. Instead of having social insurance advocates continue pushing for physician insurance, Mills decided to go ahead and incorporate it into a new Medicare plan.[44] Robert Myers, the SSA's chief actuary who worked with Mills, explains how Mills's decision came about and why he departed from his usual fidelity to fiscal conservatism to the surprise of organized labor, the Johnson administration, and the SSA:

> I remember at the close of that [executive] session when Mills leaned back and said, "Well, now, let's see. Maybe it would be a good idea if we put all three of these bills together. You (meaning the SSA) go back and work this out overnight and see what there is to this. . ."
> I think that Mills tried to put them together with the thought in mind: "Well, people have been led to believe that they are getting a lot more than just hospital benefits. And instead of having continual pressures put on us, let's broaden the scope of the program and develop it the way we want to under our own initiative, rather than under pressure from bureaucrats or the public."[45]

Mills's three-layered-cake contained something for everyone.[46] On July 27, 1965, the House passed Mills's revised bill by a margin of 307-116, and the Senate followed two days later with a 70-24 vote.[47]

With incrementalism, policymakers had finally made Social Security the logical solution. "Social Security is the only sound way of providing this type of help for our senior citizens," said Aime Forand in 1965 after Medicare's passage. "It's coming in under Social Security, and it's always easier to amend an existing law than it is to put the original law on the books."[48] Emboldened, social insurance advocates did not pause after achieving Medicare. They switched their focus from Medicare back to Social Security's engine of incrementalism, OASDI.

Changing Social Security to an Antipoverty Device

Encouraged by President Johnson's aggressive desire to fight poverty primarily through Social Security, organized labor and SSA leaders set about to transform OASDI.[49] They began in 1967 and finished with the 1972 Amendments, which incorporated: (1) an unprecedented one-time increase in benefits of 20 percent, (2) an expansion of Medicare's coverage, and (3) critical changes to OASDI's financing structure. These modifications changed the nature of Social Security and, in the process, complicated the incremental strategy for achieving universal coverage.

Prelude to the 1972 Amendments

Medicare's passage led SSA leaders, most Democrats, organized labor, and even some Republicans to continue incrementalism. The new goal became to change Social Security into an antipoverty device. The first step was OASDI benefit increases in 1967 and 1969 of 13 percent and 15 percent, respectively. Raising the taxable earnings base from $6,600 to $7,800 and the combined OASDI tax rate from 7.6 percent to 8.4 percent financed part of the increase in benefits.[50] Nevertheless, the increases were unusually large in an uncharacteristically brief period of time.[51]

Increasing OASDI benefits furthered politicians' desire to take advantage of the "electoral-economic" cycle, in which elected leaders pump up the economy in election years.[52] Johnson and Nixon were astute believers in the electoral-economic cycle as an instrument that served incumbents' reelection interests.[53] With real disposable income as the key element in the cycle, Social Security stood as the obvious tool to mail more generous checks to more people. Its annual, "unexpected" surpluses made it irresistible to presidents and congressmen hoping to use it as a political device.[54]

The unusual speed and size of benefit increases in 1967 and 1969, however, caused dissension. Some senior SSA administrators strenuously disagreed with how policymakers rationalized and justified the changes.[55] Disgusted by the ascending dominance of expansionists among Social Security's proprietors, and concerned about its effects on the overall program, Robert Myers resigned in 1970 as chief actuary for the SSA.[56] President Nixon added to Myers's disgust by deciding to retain, as commissioner of Social Security, Robert Ball (who had been appointed by Democratic President John Kennedy), instead of choosing someone more in accord with his own fiscal philosophy.[57] In resigning, Myers prophetically pointed to universal health insurance as expansionists' last, and most controversial, goal.[58]

Over time, incremental expansion of Social Security took on something of a bipartisan fervor. In January 1970, President Nixon proposed another OASDI benefit increase of 10 percent. For the first time, the House of Representatives included an amendment in its version of the legislation that would index future benefits, along with the wage base. The House did so over the vehement opposition of Ways and Means Chairman Wilbur Mills.[59] Many Republicans liked the idea because it seemingly "depoliticized" Social Security by depriving the .Democrats of credit for benefit increases. Many liberal Democrats liked it because it put the program on auto-pilot, thereby guaranteeing that benefits would stay commensurate with prices. When Congress finally passed the legislation in 1971, with indexation excluded, Nixon responded by signing the 10 percent benefit increase into law.[60] The following year, 1972, was an election year. Social Security became a leading tool in campaigns for reelection.

Passage of the 1972 Amendments

The 1967, 1969, and 1971 benefit increases, along with the 1971 advisory council's recommendations, helped to set the stage for Social Security's unprecedented changes in 1972. What emerged between partisan politics and the momentum for larger benefits was something many at the time referred to as a "bidding war."[61] Ways and Means Chairman Mills—ostensibly, but implausibly, a candidate for the Democrat's presidential nomination—came out for the largest ever benefit increase of 20 percent.[62] The 1972 amendments, which ultimately passed by overwhelming margins in Congress (302-35 in the House and 82-4 in the Senate),[63] contained a smorgasbord of structural changes and benefit increases.[64] The amendments increased benefits 20 percent and indexed (directly tied) future benefit payments and contribution rates to price and wage increases.[65] Congress assumed, therefore, that wages would rise and do so more than prices. Most important for Medicare, the amendments expanded the program to cover those receiving disability insurance and kidney dialysis.[66]

With the 1972 amendments, Social Security ceased to be conservative. The program's proprietors departed from the time-honored, ad hoc, and conservative approach of modest, incremental expansion.[67] In its place, Congress passed and the president signed the largest ever benefit increase. The average monthly check for a retired single worker jumped from $133 to $166, and from $223 to $270 for a retired couple.[68] The cumulative effect of OASI expansion between 1965 and 1975 was remarkable.[69] Monthly benefits increased 58 percent (table 5.1). Social Security benefits as a proportion of the elderly's net worth rose from one-third to one-half (table 5.2); and as a percentage of the total national income, the benefits doubled between 1965 and 1975 (table 5.3).

Table 5.1
Increases in Consumer Price Index and OASI Benefits, 1967-72

Year	CPI Increase*	OASI Benefit Increase	OASI Benefit Increase *above* CPI Increase
1967	3%	13%	10%
1969	6	15	9
1971	4	10	6
1972	6	20	14
1967-72 (total)	27^	58	31^

^ includes years not in table (CPI increase: 1968=4, 1970=4)
* rounded up

Table 5.2
Social Security as a Percentage of Elderly's Net Worth, 1955-75

Year	Social Security (in millions)	Consumers' Net Worth (in millions)	Total Worth (in millions)	Social Security as % of Total Worth
1955	$744	$1,976	$2,720	28%
1960	988	2,335	3,323	30
1965	1,507	2,645	4,152	36
1970	2,049	2,971	5,020	41
1975	3,238	3,459	6,697	49

Source: Alicia Munnell, *The Future of Social Security* (Washington, D.C.: The Brookings Institution, 1977), 118, table 6-2.

Table 5.3
OASDHI Benefits as a Percentage of Total Personal Income, 1937-80

Year	Total OASDHI Benefits (in millions)	Total Personal Income (in millions)	Total OASDHI Benefits as Percentage of Total Personal Income
1937	$1	$73,510	less than 0.05
1950	961	226,101	0.4
1960	11,245	399,724	2.8
1965	17,722	537,031	3.3
1970	38,982	801,271	4.9
1975	82,614	1,255,486	6.6
1980	156,320	2,160,975	7.0

Source: *Social Security Bulletin, Annual Statistical Supplement, 1980* (Washington, D.C.: GPO), 105.

Increasing benefits so dramatically had an immediate impact on poverty rates for the elderly: they decreased by half from 30 to 15 percent (figure 5.1). This pleased President Nixon and most members of Congress, who vastly preferred Social Security to means-tested welfare programs.

Nevertheless, the 1972 amendments shocked many in Washington because the program's generosity had never been enlarged so dramatically in so short a period.[70] "Much that was characteristic of social security policy-making was evident in the events of 1972, especially the manipulation of technique to avoid politics as conflict and to facilitate politics as the solicitation of votes," explains Martha Derthick. "Yet in some respects this event was an aberration—a departure from established norms of policy-making—and as such was profoundly disturbing to some leading participants."[71] Derthick goes on to add that the 1972 amendments, along with the benefit increases of the five preceding years, were symptomatic of a policy-making system that was disintegrating.[72]

The most significant changes to Social Security since its inception in 1935 had ramifications far beyond just the technical modifications they made to Medicare and OASDI. With the 1972 amendments, Social Security was now tied "overtly and directly to the performance of the economy."[73] The prospects for universal coverage through incremental expansion, therefore, also became largely dependent on economic circumstances.

Figure 5.1
Poverty Rate among the Elderly, 1967-73

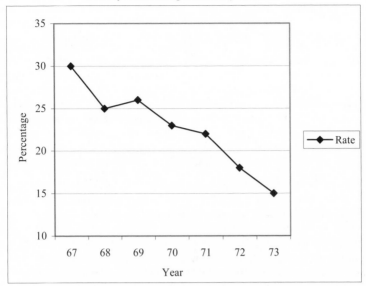

Source: U.S. Bureau of the Census, *Current Population Reports: 1979*, Series P-60
No. 130, 3.

Conclusion

During this period, health insurance gained from the strategic possibility of
being symbiotically attached to Social Security, whose popularity had been successfully secured. Policymakers' key strategy for symbiotic attachment, incrementalism, proved immensely effective. The passage of disability insurance
came first in 1956, followed by the Forand Bill in 1957 and again in 1959. The
Forand Bill failed twice, but it forced Congress to do something regarding senior
citizens' health insurance needs. Consequently, Congress passed the Kerr-Mills
program in 1960, a means-tested program for providing health insurance to the
elderly. As a joint state-federal program, though, Kerr-Mills required substantial
funding from all the individual states. This quickly proved unworkable in practice. After Kerr-Mills failed, Medicare emerged as both a logical and attractive
solution.

Modeled on the private sector's Blue Cross/Blue Shield arrangement, Medicare's structure bore testimony to the role of path dependency. Policymakers
were forced to adapt the program's design to the general form of private health
insurance. But Medicare's constituency would only be senior citizens, retirees
for the most part, which would not threaten the private path's two main constituencies and beneficiaries—employers and employees (including their dependents). Thus, Medicare reinforced the private path of tax-subsidized, employer-
provided health insurance for workers (and their dependents). It relieved active

workers of financially providing for their parents' medical needs, and then eventually became the workers' insurance provider once they reached the age of sixty-five and retired.

The public path of Social Security provided social insurance advocates opportunities they previously did not have. But the path dependency surrounding private insurance forced policymakers to conform Medicare to the structure of Blue Cross/Blue Shield, which was largely the creation of doctors and hospitals in conjunction with employers and employees. As a consequence, Medicare's political ethos mirrored the ethos of Social Security, whereas its administrative structure conformed to the existing arrangements of private health insurance.

Piggybacking Medicare onto Social Security joined the fate of universal coverage to OASDI (Social Security's cornerstone program). This was an especially promising development because of OASDI's immense popularity. Just as policymakers' use of incrementalism enabled Medicare's passage, future steps toward universal coverage could continue building on this effective strategy.

At the same time, the future success of incrementalism became more dependent than before on OASDI's popularity and financial well-being. This development partly explains why organized labor and SSA leaders so vigorously pursued major OASDI benefit increases after 1965. Already committed to the program, they now had additional incentives to pursue OASDI benefit increases. Their push for increased generosity met with great success, culminating in the Social Security Amendments of 1972. The amendments increased OASDI benefits by the biggest amount ever—20 percent. They also extended Medicare coverage to recipients of disability insurance: the first step in the program's incremental expansion down a path toward universal coverage.

Social Security's increasing complexity, with the addition of Medicare, was exacerbated by policymakers' decision to use the program as a means of fighting poverty. Congress's extension of Medicare to recipients of disability insurance in 1972, its massive OASDI benefit increases between 1967 and 1972, and the major changes it made to Social Security's wage and benefit calculations with indexation significantly reduced the program's margin for error. They explicitly tied the program to the performance of the economy. Further incremental expansion, for the purposes of reaching universal coverage, was now contingent on the economy continuing to grow sufficiently.

Notes

1. President Kennedy, among others, much preferred the slogan "Health Insurance through Social Security" to the term *Medicare*. He and other leading social insurance advocates, such as Wilbur Cohen (Department of HEW) and Nelson Cruikshank (organized labor), believed that the term *Medicare* gave the false impression that "surgical benefits" were included. Until the final version of Medicare emerged in 1965, the program proposed exclusively hospital benefits. Initially, only journalists used the term

Medicare, because it fit better in their headlines and used less print space that could otherwise go to advertising. For more explanation on this semantic predilection, see Interview with Blue Carstenson, Oral History Collection, Columbia University (1966), 94-96.

2. Theodore Marmor, *The Politics of Medicare*, 2d ed. (New York: Aldine de Gruyter, 2000), 10-11, 16-17.

3. Hugh Heclo, *Modern Social Politics in Britain and Sweden* (New Haven, Conn.: Yale University Press, 1974).

4. Paul Pierson, *Dismantling the Welfare State? Reagan, Thatcher, and the Politics of Retrenchment* (Cambridge: Cambridge University Press, 1994), 41-42. Elaborating on Heclo's observations, Paul Pierson notes how political-learning arguments focus on those actors at or near the center of the policy-making process and emphasize problems of bounded rationality or uncertainty. Policy learning theories build on research in decision-making and organizational theory, which stresses the variety of techniques used to cope with limited cognitive capacities. In effect, for policymakers, the setting of a new agenda and the design of alternative responses build on (perceived) past successes or may reflect lessons learned from past mistakes.

5. Lawrence D. Brown, "The Politics of Medicare and Health Reform, Then and Now," in *Health Care Financing Review* 18 (Winter 1996): 163.

6. Interview with Aime Forand, Oral History Collection, Columbia University (1965), 19-25. (Hereafter Forand, OHC.) Forand claims to have looked the AFL-CIO's proposal over and made several changes before agreeing to offer it as his own, but the truth is that "he never read the bill. He admitted that to us," remarked Nelson Cruikshank of the AFL-CIO. "This is a thing certainly I wouldn't want to get out. It's not fair to Aime, but it's just a matter of history. Of course Aime was not our [first] choice, not that he wasn't a good man." (Interview with Nelson Cruikshank, Oral History Collection, Columbia University [1967], 425 [Hereafter Cruikshank, OHC].

7. Interview with Allen Pond, Oral History Collection, Columbia University (1966), 44 (hereafter Pond, OHC): "I felt at that time that the Eisenhower Administration really should come up with something. I was loyal to it and trying to make it look as good as it could. And it stood for a lot of things I believed in. . . . But I felt very strongly that it had to have something that it could talk about and support. And it had nothing."

8. Forand, OHC, 25.

9. The bill's two bright spots, though, were that it increased public awareness and—at the same time—became something of a legislative martyr, which later provided political "protection" for Medicare. See Cruikshank, OHC, 441: "Politicians began to try to find a way that they could meet the need of [health insurance for the elderly] without taking on themselves the onus of supporting a thing [the Forand Bill] which had been pretty well blackened. . . . You know, the people who have said, 'I'll never vote for the Forand Bill' and 'over my dead body,' can tell their conservative constituents, 'Well, I didn't vote for the Forand Bill. I kept my promise.' But at the same time they can yield to the public pressure for something to be done. This was the kind of searching that was going on."

10. Paul Starr, *The Social Transformation of American Medicine* (New York: Basic Books, 1982), 368.

11. Interview with Elizabeth Wickenden, Oral History Collection, Columbia University (1967), 62-64. (Hereafter Wickenden, OHC.)

12. Interview with Katherine Ellickson, Oral History Collection, Columbia University (1969), 35-36, 97.

13. Wickenden, OHC, 27: "In many ways assistance is always a little bit ahead of insurance to point the way where insurance should pick up, and I don't know any place where that's clearer than in health insurance. When we come to discuss what really

helped to pass health insurance [Medicare], I would put a high priority . . . on the rising costs of medical assistance for the aged. As soon as legislators, taxpayers, and others in positions of influence became aware of the fact that for the most part they were carrying this cost anyway . . . and that it was not going to abate, there was a great advantage in finding a better way to do it."

14. See Marmor, *The Politics of Medicare*, 2d ed., 27-30. Its benefits were subject to few limits, and the federal government would provide between 50 and 80 percent of the funds. But only impoverished retirees could qualify, making it a means-tested, welfare program.

15. Interview with Robert Myers, Oral History Collection, Columbia University (1967), 36, 40 (hereafter Myers, OHC): "It was developed really as a counter-fire against the social insurance approach, just as in 1950 the APTD program, Aid to Permanently and Totally Disabled persons, was developed as a hopeful substitute to having disability benefits under social insurance. That of course didn't work either, because disability benefits were put into effect in 1956. Here, again, just about six years later, a social insurance program was put into effect because the previous public assistance program apparently hadn't filled the needs."

16. Interview with Elliot Richardson, Oral History Collection, Columbia University (1967), 42-43. Wealthier states could provide some of the necessary matching funds, but Kerr-Mills offered little help for most states that had comparatively insufficient tax revenues.

17. Cruikshank, OHC, 499.

18. See Carstenson, OHC, 47; Interview with Leonard Lesser, Oral History Collection, Columbia University (1966), 54; oblique reference in Forand, OHC, 55; and Interview with Eveline Burns, Oral History Collection, Columbia University (1965), 131: "Wilbur Mills had made this commitment to his boyfriends in Arkansas, that so long as he was Chairman of the Ways and Means Committee, no such bill was going to be released."

19. Myers, OHC, 29-30.

20. Interview with Robert Neal, Oral History Collection, Columbia University (1967), 39. Neal was a leading figure in the private insurance industry during this time.

21. Interview with Arthur Hess, Oral History Collection, Columbia University, 52-54. (Hereafter Hess, OHC).

22. Carstenson, OHC, 2-3.

23. Schorr and Lesser, OHC, 3.

24. Interview with James Brindle and Martin Cohen, Oral History Collection, Columbia University (1967), 13.

25. Cruikshank, OHC, 208: "Now, there was one other aspect to it. . . . Our public relations people . . . felt that it was not good public relations to get this battle line up as between the medical profession and organized labor. Their feeling was that if the general public is looking for guidance on a medical issue, they're not going to go to plumbers, they're going to go to doctors."

26. Carstenson, OHC, 1.

27. Schorr and Lesser, OHC, 85.

28. L. Lesser, OHC, 74-75.

29. Peter A. Corning, *The Evolution of Medicare: From Idea to Law*, Social Security Administration, Office of Research and Statistics (Washington, D.C.: GPO, 1969), 101-2.

30. Carstenson, OHC, 102-3.

31. *The Gallup Poll, Public Opinion 1935-1971*, vol. 3, 1908, 1915.

32. Cruikshank, OHC, 393-94: "If the intangible benefit of not having to submit to a means test is considered an actual benefit, then, you see, the labor people who supported the payroll tax knew jolly well that they were getting a real benefit in return for their tax. Just yesterday and this morning I had a long telephone call from an old associate of mine who, for reasons I won't go into (it's long and involved), his wife is not eligible for disability insurance. And the best I could do was to tell him to apply for welfare. He's an old labor business agent. He practically wept. He said, 'Nelson, you just don't know what you're asking me to go through. You have no idea what these people ask you about your personal life and all that, things that I'd have to reveal that I've never . . .' But people do know this. Poor people know about it. And when the working man agrees to pay a payroll tax, he's buying not just medical benefits, but he's buying his dignity and self-respect, which to him is very real and worth money."

33. Cruikshank, OHC, 393-94: "If the Social Security tax is just a tax, then it's a regressive tax, and one of the more regressive taxes. . . . But, if it is in fact an insurance premium, then it's not regressive at all. This is where that semantic difference is a real substantive difference. In fact, you see, it's less regressive than a private insurance premium. If a working man takes out a $5,000 life insurance policy, he pays exactly the same rate on it, if he's making $4,000 a year as his $100,000 a year boss pays on a $5,000 life insurance policy, assuming they're the same age and in the same health condition—in other words, assuming they're covering the same risk. However, under Social Security, the working man pays a lesser rate than the higher paid man. So, as insurance it's the least regressive of the insurance premiums in America."

34. Hess, OHC, 74.

35. Hess, OHC, 86-87: "Although much of our planning went along 100% federal lines originally, I think it was politically unrealistic, and it became clear that one way to calm the fears of hospital people, and one way to have a proposal in the Congress that had a minimum amount of political viability, was in effect to say, 'Well, you'll be dealing with the same people that you deal with every day on the same kind of payment basis, so there'll be nothing strange about this. The day-to-day administration will be in the hands of persons who you know and who have the know-how and procedures and policies and so on to reimburse hospitals in a way that hospitals get reimbursed in any third-party payment system.' In effect, we were reducing the degree of change and reducing the potential for fear and opposition in the legislative process and for disruption in the operation."

36. Cruikshank, OHC, 249-50.

37. Theodore Marmor, *The Politics of Medicare* (Chicago: Aldine Publishing Company, 1973). For more on the political history of Medicare, see: E. Feingold, *Medicare: Policy and Politics* (San Francisco: Chandler, 1966), ch. 3; Richard Harris, *A Sacred Trust* (New York: New American Library, 1966); James L. Sundquist, *Politics and Policy: The Eisenhower, Kennedy, and Johnson Years* (Washington, D.C.: Brookings Institution, 1968), 287-322; Sheri I. David, *With Dignity: The Search for Medicare and Medicaid*; Max Skidmore, *Medicare and the American Rhetoric of Reconciliation* (University, Ala.: University of Alabama Press, 1970); and Peter A. Corning, *The Evolution of Medicare: From Idea to Law*, U.S. Department of Health, Education, and Welfare: Social Security Administration, Office of Research and Statistics (Washington, D.C.: GPO, 1969).

38. Corning, *The Evolution of Medicare*, 112.

39. Transcript, Wilbur Mills History Interview II (March 25, 1987), by Michael L. Gillette, electronic copy, LBJ Library, 2-3.

40. Transcript, Mills, 4.

41. Transcript, Mills, 4.

42. Martha Derthick, *Policymaking for Social Security* (Washington, D.C.: The Brookings Institution, 1979), 331.

43. Medicaid, Medicare's means-tested companion for the poor, in some ways was also a beneficiary of the successful strategy of incrementalism, because the program passed through the same window of opportunity that Medicare did. But because Medicaid never gained the permanent status of "entitlement," the program was an unlikely stepping-stone for reaching universal coverage. Instead, Medicare was the key step upon which policymakers hoped to build. Moreover, Medicaid quickly acquired the stigma of "second-class" medical care, because its reimbursement rates were so low by the industry's standards. As a noncontributory welfare scheme, therefore, Medicaid gained far more from the incremental success that OASDI made possible than it returned in political capital to those pursuing additional expansions of social insurance.

44. Transcript, Wilbur Mills Oral History Interview (November 2, 1971), by Joe B. Frantz, electronic copy, LBJ Library, 11.

45. Myers, OHC, 91. Confirmed by Arthur Hess in personal interview with the author (December 18, 1997).

46. Organized labor was not particularly fond of Medicare's final structure (particularly Part B), as Lee Bamberger of the AFL-CIO told an interviewer: "I think it was a very ingenious way of dealing with the opposition and dealing with a lot of problems that involved ingenious dealing and manipulation and operation at high levels, which I think was very appealing as a way of solving [several political] problems. This one really had a tremendous elegance about it, this three-layered cake. There's a great beauty in terms of the political machinations involved. And the fact that it wasn't really substantively elegant I think became secondary. I think that therefore there was a great stake in our [organized labor] not looking too closely at it. There was also in the general atmosphere the whole business that you were not supposed to be a soft or a muddle-headed liberal, where you raise a lot of programmatic issues all the time, that you have to be a hard-headed pragmatist and you have to figure out what works. . . .

[W]e had finally trapped the Republicans. . . . The AMA had run these ads on how inadequate Medicare was—it doesn't do this, it doesn't do this, it doesn't do this—and now we had a program that did all these things. And nobody could be against it" (Schorr and Lesser, OHC, 29-30).

47. Marmor, *The Politics of Medicare*, 1st ed., 74.

48. Forand, OHC, 21-23.

49. See Julian Zelizer, *Taxing America: Wilbur D. Mills, Congress, and the State, 1945-1975* (Cambridge: Cambridge University Press, 1998), ch. 10, 312-46.

50. *Social Security Bulletin* 31 (February 1968): 3 and 36 (March 1973): 4.

51. For account of 1967-69 benefit increases, see Derthick, *Policymaking for Social Security*, 339-49.

52. See Edward R. Tufte, *Political Control of the Economy* (Princeton: Princeton University Press, 1978).

53. See Walter Heller, *New Dimensions of Political Economy* (Cambridge: Harvard University Press, 1966), 12; and Richard M. Nixon, *Six Crises* (Garden City, N.Y.: Doubleday, 1962), 309-11.

54. Derthick, *Policymaking for Social Security*, 348: Social Security's actuarial "estimates were made on the assumption that earnings would remain level. When earnings rose—as they invariably did—an actuarial surplus was 'discovered.'"

55. Edward Berkowitz, *Mr. Social Security: The Life of Wilbur Cohen* (Lawrence: University Press of Kansas, 1995), 290.

56. Zelizer, *Taxing America*, 326-27.

57. Edward Berkowitz, *America's Welfare State* (Baltimore: Johns Hopkins University Press, 1991), 69.

58. Robert Myers, *Expansionism in Social Insurance* (London: Institute of Economic Affairs, 1970), 22: "The ultimate goal of the expansionists in medical care is relatively simple, but comprehensive: to provide 'Medicare' benefits for the entire working and retired populations and their dependents. . . . Once again, the expansionists would take the gradual approach to their desired social goal. This would be done by first extending Medicare for some or all of the persons under age 65 who are receiving cash benefits. Then, there might be instituted the so-called 'Kiddiecare' proposal. . . . Certainly the consequence of establishing a Kiddiecare program would be to reduce further the potential scope of private insurance. As a result, the relative operating costs of private insurance for the limited benefit area in which it would operate would become high. Private insurance would thus be subject to adverse criticism, and it would be suggested that the governmental plan might as well take over the entire load since it could operate more efficiently from an administrative point."

59. Zelizer, *Taxing America*, 324-26.

60. Robert Ball, "Social Security Amendments of 1972: Summary and Legislative History," *Social Security Bulletin* 36 (March 1973): 5-11.

61. The term *bidding war* has been used by many to describe the events surrounding the 1972 OASDI legislation, including by President George Bush's director of the Office of Management and Budget, Richard Darman, who was a staff member at the Department of HEW in 1972: "I have fond memories from my early days at HEW in the late sixties and early seventies when I was associated with the then Cabinet Committee on Aging. It was a lot more fun in those days, if I may say, because we were figuring out how to expand benefits under every heading, and we were not too concerned about costs. As I know you and other members of the Committee will recall well, at one point we got into a bidding war on Social Security and ultimately passed the 20 percent Social Security benefit increase, which had a very favorable effect on the income position of older Americans." As quoted in "Medicare and Medicaid Budget Priorities in the 1990's," *Hearings before the Select Committee on Aging,* House of Representatives, 101st Congress, 1st Session (March 23, 1989), 21.

62. Zelizer, *Taxing America*, 331-37.

63. "20% Social Security Rise Is Voted by Both Houses," *New York Times*, July 1 1972, 1.

64. For comprehensive discussion of the changes produced by the 1972 Amendments, see Ball, "Social Security Amendments of 1972," 3-23. For detailed explanation of how the 1972 amendments came about, see Derthick, *Policymaking for Social Security*, 349-68.

65. R. Kent Weaver, *Automatic Government: The Politics of Indexation* (Washington, D.C.: The Brookings Institution, 1988).

66. For elaboration, see Robert Myers, *Medicare* (Bryn Mawr, Pa.: McCahan Foundation, 1970), 64-72.

67. Weaver, *Automatic Government*, 79.

68. Andrew Achenbaum, *Social Security: Visions and Revisions* (Cambridge: Cambridge University Press, 1986), 58.

69. See Robert Ball, *Social Security Today and Tomorrow* (New York: Columbia University Press, 1978), 18-19.

70. Derthick, *Policymaking for Social Security*, 365-68.

71. Zelizer, *Taxing America*, 344-46.

Chapter Five

72. Derthick, *Policymaking for Social Security*, 365.
73. Derthick, *Policymaking for Social Security*, 368.

CHAPTER SIX

Incrementalism's Consequences

Rising Costs, Narrowing Paths
(1970s)

Nineteen months ago I said that America's medical system faced a "massive crisis."
Since that statement was made, that crisis has deepened. All of us must now join together
in a common effort to meet this crisis—each of us doing his part to mobilize more effec-
tively the enormous potential of our health care system.

—President Richard Nixon (1971)

Social insurance advocates were convinced that incrementalism was the best strategy for achieving universal coverage.[1] They pointed logically to Medicare as the first major step in a series that would eventually result in universal coverage. Robert Ball, Social Security's commissioner from 1962 to 1973, finally admitted in 1996—despite numerous earlier denials—that incrementalism was indeed the covert strategy for achieving universal health insurance coverage:

A first step toward universal coverage: For people who are trying to understand what we were up to, the first broad point to keep in mind is that all of us who developed Medicare and fought for it—including Nelson Cruikshank of the AFL-CIO and Wilbur Cohen, . . . myself and others at the Social Security Administration—had been advocates of universal national health insurance. We and the principals for whom we worked—George Meany, the AFL-CIO president, Social Security Commissioner Arthur Altmeyer, and others—had become discouraged about the prospects of enacting universal health insurance as such.

We saw insurance for the elderly as a fallback position, which we advocated solely because it seemed to have the best chance politically. Although the public record contains some explicit denials, we expected Medicare to be a first step toward universal health insurance, perhaps with "Kiddiecare" as another step.[2]

Instead of leading to further steps, though, Medicare precipitated a sharp escalation in the costs of medical care.[3] As experience mounted, so did obstacles to further enactments. Medicare ran into financial trouble in its first decade of operation for two reasons: its immediate availability to all senior citizens,[4] and its integration into Social Security. Policymakers' decision to integrate Medicare into Social Security transformed the health insurance program into an "efficient claims payment" operation lacking effective cost containment.[5]

Medicare's financial escalation occurred at a disadvantageous time, because during the 1970s the United States came closer than ever before to attaining universal coverage through a national health insurance program.[6] Prospects for the goal improved substantially when Richard Nixon presented the first national health insurance proposal by a Republican president in 1971. Resubmitting a modified version of his plan in 1974, he designated it his "number one, major initiative on the domestic policy agenda."[7] Even the AMA, long the archenemy of national health insurance, had its own proposal for universal coverage called "Medicredit." National health insurance appeared to be, in Nixon's own words, "an idea whose time had come in America."[8]

In reviewing the failed strategies and legislative outcomes of the 1970s, we are left with two questions. Why did Medicare fail to culminate in universal coverage? And with so much in its favor, what defeated national health insurance in 1974?

This chapter argues that policymakers' design and implementation of Medicare led to an acutely damaging cost explosion. By the time a window of opportunity for national health insurance opened in 1974, the program's public path had narrowed dramatically (if not closed) for the purposes of incremental expansion. Emerging concerns over Social Security's solvency[9] damaged Medicare's capacity to carry program development down a fruitful path, because it contributed to Ways and Means members' perception that Social Security's payroll tax was too high to support any expansion.[10] By 1977, Dan Rostenkowski, chairman of the Ways and Means Subcommittee on Health, was telling reporters that higher Social Security taxes dimmed the chances for national health insurance.[11]

At the same time, exiting to new paths for achieving universal coverage was also impossible, in part because organized labor refused to compromise its demand for pure national health insurance. The fact that labor advocated exiting to a public path initially seems counterintuitive. Yet despite labor's remarkable success at collectively bargaining for health insurance during the 1950s and 1960s, it also had a larger philosophical tradition of advocating pure social insurance dating back to the early 1940s. Labor temporarily subordinated its commitment to national health insurance because collective bargaining proved so effective in securing private protection for workers and their families (in the form of fringe benefits). This success quickly spilled over into the vast majority of nonunionized workers as well.

But the success policymakers finally had in passing Medicare in 1965, together with the rampant medical inflation it subsequently generated, contributed to labor's decision to revert to its traditional position of insisting on a public approach modeled on (if not directly attached to) Social Security. In the early 1970s, labor gambled that it could do to health insurance what Franklin Roosevelt and his successors eventually did to pensions—make it publicly universal.

Medicare's Failure to Further Program Development

The addition of Medicare, along with benefit increases in the basic program (OASDI), changed the nature of Social Security from providing an adequate minimum protection for those most at risk, the elderly, to maintaining a standard of relative comfort.[12] This metamorphosis had been an objective of many of the programs' founders from the start. But it benefited in some measure from a growing perception in the 1960s that Social Security was undoubtedly the most successful program developed by any modern welfare state. "[It] is squarely based on the 8th wonder of the world—compound interest," Paul Samuelson, the country's foremost economist, brazenly claimed in 1967. "A growing nation is the greatest Ponzi game ever contrived. And that is a fact, not a paradox."[13]

Social Security was indeed a "most successful program," as Samuelson said, but it was also a program limited exclusively to retirees, survivors, and the disabled. This created various gaps in people's coverage over the course of their lives.[14] Consequently, social insurance advocates sought to change Social Security from a largely age-based safety-net program to a broader, more generous scheme of lifetime insurance. Their strategy of choice, Wilbur Cohen explained, amounted to a continuation of incremental expansion:

> The cyclical change in power ushers in a new era. But irrespective of rhetoric, philosophy, . . . or political leadership, the only option open is to build upon the past. Change it here and there; add something; change its name; cut off some fuzzy edges; and then proclaim the new day is here in which a new approach has been unveiled to overcome the mistakes of the past.[15]

Cohen's assertion assumed that economic growth would continue more or less in the same manner it had since 1945. Recessions would come and go, but the basic pattern would be growth in wages that outstripped growth in prices.[16]

As long as this stable economic pattern of growth continued and the birth rate remained relatively stable, what could thwart Social Security's expansionary growth? As it turns out, two things in particular: (1) broadening Social Security from cash benefits to include medical insurance in the form of Medicare, and (2) dramatically increasing and indexing OASDI benefits in a short period of time, 1967-72. Medicare's profligacy, together with the effects of OASDI's large benefit increases between 1967 and 1972, converged in the mid-1970s to the shock of nearly everyone. Medicare insolvency warnings arose in the first decade after its implementation. Long-term financial threats to OASDI surfaced for the first time in 1973, and short-term threats by 1974.[17] The latter prompted the image of Social Security in "crisis." Most important, Medicare and OASDI's cost explosion tarnished the overall image of Social Security, and, in the process, crippled incrementalism.

Medicare's Profligacy

Medicare's lack of cost control proved damaging to its credibility.[18] By 1972, even social insurance enthusiasts agreed that Medicare's "victory" had come at great expense. In trying to avoid the wrath of the medical community, Congress passed Medicare with few cost controls.[19] The program quickly became a generous "claims payment" operation for doctors and hospitals. Its popularity grew quickly, but at the expense of cost containment.[20] While the SSA could reasonably predict the costs of Social Security's OASDI cash benefits program, it had practically no way to reliably estimate—much less control—expenditures.[21] Social insurance supporters admitted this at the seventh Social Security Conference in Ann Arbor, Michigan, in April 1972:

> *Wilbur Cohen*: Should restructuring have come first [with Medicare]?
>
> *Melvin Glasser, UAW*: Well, there are two answers. You know the first better than I, because in the Medicare legislation passed in your administration (not at your wish, but nonetheless there it was) there is language to this effect: "Nothing in this bill shall do anything to change the present method of delivery of services." The American people and you as an administrator were locked in. There's nothing you could do; you were prohibited from changing the delivery system.
>
> The second aspect is that restructuring is needed. . . . You can't deal with a piece of the system, as Medicare has found. You can't change the way a hospital delivers services, for example, when only 20 percent of its patients, and somewhere around 20 percent of its income, comes from Medicare.[22]

Policymakers knew that Medicare lacked adequate cost controls. Wilbur Cohen admitted as much: "The sponsors of Medicare, including myself, had to concede in 1965 that there would be no real controls over hospitals and physicians. I was required to promise before the final vote in the Executive Session of the House Ways and Means Committee that the Federal agency would exercise no control."[23] Lacking sufficient cost-control mechanisms, Medicare's expenditures quickly became a problem.[24] President Johnson fumed in 1967 that Wilbur Mills was "all over the ticker" in his attempt to explain Medicare's increased costs.[25] In 1974, Mills admitted that Medicare's costs had increased far beyond the original estimates, largely because no provisions for cost containment existed.[26] By 1980, four years after his departure from Congress, Mills was candid about the program's financial escalation:

You know, when you author a program, you expect it to be perfect. I thought Medicare was. I thought it would take care of the costs of the medical problems that older citizens would encounter. We never envisioned anything such as we are hearing today of the . . . total costs that are being paid by this program.[27]

Medicare's problems with cost control were essentially the result of what Theodore Marmor and Paul Starr have referred to as the program's "politics of accommodation."[28] In attempting to gain the cooperation of doctors and hospitals, the Social Security Administration's approach to running Medicare demonstrated three "accommodating" characteristics: (1) a commitment to remaining primarily a distributor of popular entitlement benefits, (2) a desire to avoid controversy and have operations run smoothly, and (3) an effort to secure exclusive administration of Medicare.[29] "The strategy was eminently successful in getting Medicare under way and accepted," argues Judith Feder. "But in the process, maintaining the compromises through which the goal was achieved became an end in itself."[30]

One result of the SSA's desire to have the medical community embrace Medicare was that doctors' "prevailing, customary, and reasonable" fees—the criteria by which the program based its remuneration—rose precipitously (table 6.1). Young doctors began billing at unprecedented levels and the SSA paid them. When older doctors saw the behavior of their younger associates, they, too, raised their fees.[31]

Table 6.1
Annual Percentage Increase in CPI and Medical Care, 1955-70

Inflation in	(pre-Medicare) 1955-60	(pre-Medicare) 1960-65	(post-Medicare) 1965-70	Percentage Higher Than CPI (1965-70)
CPI	2.0%	1.3%	4.2%	—
All Medical Care	4.1	2.5	6.1	45%
Hospital Charges	6.3	5.8	13.9	231
Physicians' Fees	3.3	2.8	6.6	57

Source: "Medical Care Expenditures, Prices and Costs: Background Book," Social Security Administration, DHEW Pub. No. (SSA) 74-11909, 25, table 2.

Although doctors' demands became a major cause of Medicare's profligacy, physician costs paled in comparison to those of hospitals.[32] "Medicare gave hospitals a license to spend," according to Rosemary Taylor. "The more expenditures they incurred, the more income they received. Medicare tax funds flowed into hospitals in a golden stream, more than doubling between 1970 and 1975, and doubling again by 1980."[33] Medicare's formula for hospital reimbursement invited abuse, because it operated on a "cost+ 2 percent basis" for all services. Since the 2 percent was a percentage of costs, it amounted to an open-ended proposition by offering a small bonus for every cost increase. So while the CPI increased 89 percent between 1966 and 1976, hospital costs grew a staggering

345 percent.[34] In effect, medical providers took advantage of the unique economic dynamics surrounding medical care: Although the occurrence of illness
usually exists beyond one's control, the demand for care constitutes essentially a
discretionary decision. Insurance against the financial costs of health services,
such as Medicare, allows the consumption of those services to vastly increase
(tables 6.1, 6.2).[35]

Table 6.2
Hospital Costs, 1955-76

Year	Average Annual Percentage Increase In Cost per Patient-day	Percentage Increase from Period Before	Average Annual Percentage Increase in Cost per Patient-day^	Percentage Increase from Period Before
1955-60	6.9	—	5.9	—
1960-66	7.0	1%	5.3	-10%
1966-71†	14.1	101	9.0	70
1971-74*	11.5	-19	4.4	-51
1974-76	16.9	47	8.7	98

Source: Adapted and modified from Martin Feldstein, *Hospital Costs and Health Insurance*
        (Cambridge, Mass.: Harvard University Press, 1981), 22.
* Wage and price controls in effect
^ Relative to consumer price index (CPI)
† First five years of Medicare

Table 6.3
Medicare Costs in Billions, Parts A and B, 1967-95

Year	Total Costs	Part A (Hospital)	Percentage Increase	Part B (Physician)	Percentage Increase
1967	$4.6	$3.4	—	$1.2	—
1970	7.1	5.1	50	2.0	67
1975	15.6	11.3	123	4.3	115
1980	35.7	25.1	122	10.6	147
1985	70.5	47.6	90	22.9	116
1990	108.7	66.2	39	42.5	86
1995	181.4	116.4	76	65.0	53

Source: Board of Trustees, Federal Hospital Insurance Trust Fund, 1996.

Because Medicare lacked sufficient financial restraint, cost estimates soon
fell glaringly short of initial predictions.[36] When Congress passed Medicare in
1965, the House Ways and Means Committee projected annual expenditures of
$238 million. Assuming that 95 percent of the elderly might enroll in Part B—
this prediction proved accurate—the committee estimated that, at most, total
Medicare costs would be $1.3 billion in 1967, the first full year of operation.[37]
The cost, instead, came in at $4.6 billion. The committee also predicted hospital
insurance expenses to be $3.1 billion for 1970 and $4.2 billion for 1975, with
money left over in the hospital trust fund. Actual costs were $7.1 billion and
$15.6 billion, respectively.[38] Medicare expenditures doubled every five years
until 1990 (table 6.3).

Unlike OASDI's costs, which remained misleadingly low for decades, Medicare's costs exploded quickly.[39] The manner in which Congress inaugurated the program partly explains why.[40] Basically, it immediately "blanketed in" 19 million beneficiaries on July 1, 1966, without any of them ever having paid into the program. Medicare's structure precluded it from experiencing a "grace" period in which its trust funds could build up some measure of reserves from modest annual surpluses.[41] Instead, as Jonathan Oberlander has documented, Medicare began operation as a genuine "pay as you go" system.[42] Active workers initially paid for retirees' hospital benefits through their payroll taxes for Part A, and for retirees' physician benefits through their general income taxes for Part B. Participants' monthly contributions helped with Part B, but over time they covered less and less of the program's costs.[43]

Finally, Medicare made all medical care more expensive (see table 6.4), significantly increasing it as a share of the country's GNP. In the fifteen years before Medicare's passage, health expenditures as a percentage of GNP increased 31 percent. In the fifteen years after its passage, their share increased by 53 percent. When Medicare passed, total health expenditures were $38.9 billion per year and 5.9 percent of GNP. By 1980, this figure had increased an astonishing 535 percent to $247.2 billion per year and 9 percent of GNP—the world's highest.[44] Of course, the rising costs of health care were not solely Medicare's fault. Yet the increase in national expenditures (29 percent) for health care in the five years following the program's implementation is incommensurably higher than any other five-year period before or after (table 6.4; see also table 6.2).

In other words, Medicare produced an expenditure spike that permeated the country's entire medical system. Even after the spike subsided, large cost increases continued (table 6.4). As a result, Oberlander explains, Medicare "acquired a negative reputation among political elites. That negative reputation diminished the political viability of Medicare as a model for national health insurance."[45]

Table 6.4
Total Health Expenditures as a Percentage of GNP, 1960-80

Year	Total Health Expenditures (billions)	Percentage Increase	Expenditures as Percentage of GNP	Percentage Increase
1960	$26.9	—	5.2	—
1965	38.9	45	5.9	13
1970^	74.7	92	7.6	29
1975*	131.5	76	8.6	13
1980	247.2	88	9.0	5

Source: Adapted and modified from Robert M. Gibson, "National Health Expenditures, 1978," *Health Care Financing Review* 1 (Summer 1979), tables 1, 3; *The 1981 Budget in Brief*, Executive Office of the President, 48.
^ Expenditure spike in first five years of Medicare's existence
* Wage and price controls in effect 1971-74

National Health Insurance: The Missed Opportunity

Medicare's cost spike contributed to a rise in public pressure for health care reform in the early 1970s. According to Republican Senator Jacob Javits of New York, "One unexpected result of Medicare was a sharp increase in medical costs for all Americans, which revived interest in a comprehensive system of health insurance to cover everyone."[46]

Arguably, 1974 stands out as the closest that comprehensive national health insurance has ever come to fruition in the United States. "If ever there were a year in which NHI had a serious chance of being adopted," as Flint Wainess has shown, "it was 1974."[47] In late 1973, the *Atlantic Monthly* argued that "some kind of national health insurance has seemed in recent years to be an idea whose time has finally come in America."[48] President Nixon resubmitted a modified version of his 1971 proposal for national health insurance on January 19, 1974.[49] In the same year, the *New York Times* editorialized that "much potential waste could readily be avoided by use of the Social Security system as the basic insurance mechanism" for a comprehensive health insurance program.[50] The *Washington Post* also editorialized that "the parade of witnesses has shown clearly that the question being debated is not whether the United States should have national health insurance, but what kind it should be."[51] *Newsweek* magazine concurred: "The fact remains that national health insurance at last seems an idea whose time has come—and that many of those who have most bitterly opposed the idea in the past seem prepared to go along with some version of the two major proposals now under discussion."[52] Alice Rivlin entitled an article in the *New York Times Magazine* in the summer of 1974, "Agreed: Here Comes National Health Insurance."[53] Even Wilbur Mills proclaimed that "health insurance will pass by October 1."[54] Optimism, which began increasing in 1971, had reached an all-time high.

"From Medicare to National Health Insurance,"[55] First Try in 1971

Ideological cleavages over the issue of national health insurance appeared to have dissipated by the early 1970s. The ordinarily hostile AMA proposed its first-ever plan for national health insurance in 1971 called "Medicredit" (tax credits for health insurance) that competed with the first-ever plan offered by a Republican president, Richard Nixon. Nixon's proposal in 1971, the "National Health Insurance Partnership," was something of a compromise between the AMA's voluntary Medicredit plan and organized labor's Health Security Act. Nixon's National Health Insurance Partnership, as Marie Gottschalk has detailed, mandated that employers purchase insurance for their workers.[56] Many critics dismiss Nixon's national health insurance proposals as "Disraeli Tory Reformism" (stealing progressive issues from partisan opponents for political gain, while not genuinely pursuing them). But Nixon's national health insurance speech to Congress on February 18, 1971, two years before the extraordinary pressures of Watergate came to bear on him and his administration, suggests that scholars ought to be careful before rushing to accuse Nixon of opportunism:

For growing numbers of Americans, the cost of care is becoming prohibitive. Even those who can afford most care may find themselves impoverished by a catastrophic medical expenditure. The quality of medicine varies widely with geography and income. . . . Costs have skyrocketed but values have not kept pace. We are investing more of our nation's resources in the health of our people, but we are not getting a full return on our investment.

Too many health insurance policies focus on hospital and surgical costs and leave critical outpatient services uncovered. Because demand goes where the dollars are, the result is an unnecessary—and expensive—over-utilization of acute care facilities. A second problem is the failure of most private insurance policies to protect against the catastrophic costs of major illnesses and accidents. This means that insurance often runs out while expenses are still mounting. For many of our families, the anguish of a serious illness is thus compounded by acute financial anxiety. Even the joy of recovery can often be clouded by the burden of debt—and even by the threat of bankruptcy.

I am proposing that a National Health Insurance Standards Act be adopted which will require employers to provide basic health insurance for their employees. In the past, we have taken similar actions to assure workers a minimum wage, to provide them with disability and retirement benefits and to set occupational health and safety standards. Now we should go one step further and guarantee that all workers will receive adequate health insurance protection. The federal government would pay nothing for this program: the costs would be shared by employers and employees, much as they are today under most collective bargaining agreements.

I am also proposing that a new Family Health Insurance Plan be established to meet the special needs of poor families. Medicaid suffers from defects that now plague our failing welfare system. It largely excludes the working poor—which means that all benefits can suddenly be cut off when a family's income rises ever so slightly. Coverage is provided when husbands desert their families, but is often eliminated when they come back home and work. Some of these problems would be corrected by my proposal to require employers to offer adequate insurance coverage to their employees. No longer, for example, would a working man receive poorer insurance coverage than a welfare client—a condition that exists today in many states.

"It is health which is real worth," said Gandhi, "and not pieces of gold and silver." That statement applies not only to the lives of men but also to the life of nations. Not only is health more important than economic wealth, it is also its foundation. Nineteen months ago I said that America's medical system faced a "massive crisis." Since that statement was made, that crisis has deepened. All of us must now join together in a common effort to meet this crisis—each doing his own part to mobilize more effectively the enormous potential of our health care system.[57]

Organized labor opposed Nixon's bill because it maintained a primary role for private insurance carriers, and because it competed against labor's Health Security Act. Employers (particularly small and seasonal businesses) opposed it because it imposed new regulations and requirements. Private insurance carriers remained indifferent, neither opposing nor supporting Nixon's plan.[58]

The three proposals in 1971 defined the debate's parameters. Labor's Health Security Act marked the liberal end of the spectrum, the AMA's Medicredit the conservative end, and Nixon's National Health Insurance Partnership the middle ground. Although the plans' details varied widely, all of them voiced public support for universal health insurance coverage. Compromise appeared imminent and necessary.

Organized labor's insistence on a public approach appeared to run counter to its vested interest in health insurance's private path, but the advent of Medicare permanently altered its preferences. With the program's passage in 1965 serving as a possible stepping-stone, labor reverted to its long-standing philosophical commitment to the larger goal of universal national health insurance.[59] At the same time, the inflationary cost spike that Medicare produced led to labor's increased frustration with collective bargaining. The health insurance component of union contracts failed to keep pace with rising prices, so workers' out-of-pocket costs continued to rise. The AFL-CIO's George Meany wrote in 1970:

> Many unions have found that they have been on a sort of treadmill. . . . Just as fast as we could negotiate money to provide more and better health services for our members, the doctors raised their fees and the hospitals boosted their charges. Thus, in health care, we have a very unusual situation which we don't like at all. . . . We have had a pretty good record in collective bargaining of getting more money for health care. But instead of making our members and their families better off through more comprehensive health services, we have simply been making more money for doctors.[60]

Labor's frustration, coupled with its belief that the political environment in the early 1970s was more auspicious than it had ever been, led union leadership in Washington to single-mindedly pursue its most utopian vision of medical provision: pure national health insurance. Labor's position represented an eagerness on its part to abandon the private path, but *only* for the one scenario it had always considered superior, the public path of social insurance. Essentially, organized labor wanted a health insurance program similar to Social Security: universal, comprehensive, and untouched by inflation, three characteristics that their private, collectively bargained plans lacked.[61] Senator Edward Kennedy submitted labor's Health Security Act in 1971.[62]

As advertised by the AFL-CIO, the structure of labor's plan bore testimony to the interest group's desire for pure social insurance: "Health Security is a national system—just as Social Security is a national system."[63] Labor repeatedly emphasized Health Security's relation to Social Security with its ethos of benefits by right because of beneficiaries' contributions: "The tried, proven and accepted method of Social Security taxes would provide half the revenue needed [for the Health Security Act]. Employers, employees and the self-employed would contribute to the Health Security Trust Fund on this basis: employers, 3.5 percent of payroll; self-employed, 2.5 percent of income up to $15,000; employees and others, 1 percent of income up to $15,000."[64]

One of the most revealing glimpses of labor's position came during the House Ways and Means Committee's hearings on the issue in 1971, in an exchange between Democratic member Omar Burleson (Tex.) and the UAW's Leonard Woodcock:

Burleson: Mr. Woodcock, let me ask you this: Would you consider H.R. 22 [Health Security Act] to be a nationalization of the health industry generally?

Woodcock: No, sir. It is a partnership of a national financing scheme just like the social security system. . . .

Burleson: Of course, social security didn't replace anything. It came into being on its own without the massive effort called for in this type of legislation.

Woodcock: This is not a copying of the British or Soviet system or any other system. It starts by building on the system as it is and . . . moving toward a more efficient system.

Burleson: But to remove an industry like the insurance industry completely from health care . . . is a radical departure from what we have. I can't see where there is a very great partnership in your recommendations. . . . I am speaking of insurance as being a facet of the entire health industry—the medical profession itself. . . . Anyway I just can't imagine that the Government is designed for this sort of thing. . . . [T]he Government could not efficiently run such a program.

Woodcock: Well, there is one program that is operating exceedingly well. Its benefits are too low for the social good, but the social security system to which this is most analogous is operating very successfully.

Burleson: Yes, I think so. I would agree to that, but it didn't supplant something that we had before. We had insurance, of course, for retirement, annuities in industry and labor and other parts of our society that it did not supplant. But it was something for people who didn't have that sort of coverage.[65]

The 1971 hearings on national health insurance did not lead to any substantive action. The Ways and Means Committee failed to report a bill. And Nixon moved away from his original proposal, choosing instead to focus his administration's energies on "a new health strategy" involving health maintenance organizations (HMOs).[66] So the moment passed and the issue of universal coverage receded.

Second Try: 1974

A renewed push for national health insurance in early 1974 coincided with rapidly increasing medical costs that followed the expiration of wage and price controls.[67] "It appears that the right combination of forces might break the stalemate which had prevented enactment of health insurance legislation for 30 years," wrote *CQ Weekly*.[68] "The administration has been pushing for action in 1974 and talking compromise. Key congressional Democrats have agreed that the time has come to act and indicated that they, too, were ready to make some compromises."[69] The Ways and Means Committee and Senate Finance Committee opened the first legislative hearings on health insurance in three years.[70]

The ending of President Nixon's "Economic Stabilization Program" made cost containment as important as universal coverage.[71] Universal coverage remained a top priority, but limiting health care expenditures became the clarion call. Thus, the strategy of incrementalism became increasingly complicated.

As in 1949 and 1971, the lack of agenda-setting control in 1974 led to a debilitating proliferation of plans for national health insurance.[72] Once interest groups sensed that comprehensive reform was likely, they flooded Congress with alternative proposals.[73] Seven health insurance programs eventually competed against each other in 1974, four of which observers considered to be major contenders (table 6.5): the AMA's Medicredit, Nixon's modified Comprehensive Health Insurance Act, Kennedy-Mills's compromise National Health Insurance Act, and the original, labor-supported Health Security Act.[74]

Ironically, although it traditionally had the greatest interest in this type of legislation, organized labor was the *only* interest group that refused to compromise: "We have evaluated these proposals," said the AFL-CIO, "and we state unequivocally that the Health Security Bill is the only proposal before the Congress which meets these principles."[75] Labor even admitted that it wanted no bill if the Health Security proposal could not pass. According to AFL-CIO spokesman Allen Zack, "We had to take too much insurance industry involvement in Medicare. We learned a lot from that. It's a matter of rushing through a bad bill, and we don't want it."[76]

The AFL-CIO responded to criticism by Senator Kennedy and others seeking a compromise by stating that it would prefer to wait a year if need be, "when Congress may be more liberal."[77] Labor's intransigence was most clearly revealed in a confrontational exchange between members of the Ways and Means Committee and Andy Biemiller, director of the AFL-CIO's Department of Legislation:

Congressman Burleson, D-TX: Mr. Biemiller, your attitude is unless you get the full adoption of that measure [the Health Security Act], you would prefer that there be no bill at all in this session. . . . Is that your attitude?

Mr. Biemiller: What we have said is that we do not think that any of the bills that are being offered as a compromise bill, including Mills-Kennedy, meet the basic principles that we think ought to go into a sound health insurance bill.

We have not forgotten, for example, . . . that in 1964 the Congress did not want to pass any kind of a Medicare bill. A big flap went on over the fact and, as a result, a bill that would have increased social security benefits got held up and did not pass in 1964.

By the time 1965 came around, many of those who had fought Medicare very hard had become advocates of Medicare, and we have a feeling that the same kind of thing can prevail with national insurance. . . .

Congressman Clancy, R-OH: Mr. Biemiller, [you're saying that] organized labor is not going to approve of any national health program this year short of [the Health Security Act], because labor feels that the climate next year will be much better to get what it wants. Now, is that a fact?

Mr. Biemiller: As I stated earlier, . . . the years 1964-65 demonstrated to us pretty effectively that we do gain sometimes by having to delay for a year or so the enactment of legislation.[78]

After labor's testimony before Congress, the *Washington Post* scolded labor in an editorial: "Labor's leadership should stop painting its utopias with a broad brush and get into the practical realistic debate that is taking place on Capitol Hill right now. With union support, a comprehensive bill preserving the best features of the Kennedy-Mills approach would stand a good chance of passage."[79]

Organized labor ignored criticism of its rigid stance and stiffened its resolve, convinced that 1974 was, politically speaking, the same as 1964.[80] Labor thought that waiting a year until after the 1964 elections had led to an improved Medicare bill in 1965 compared with the original Senate-passed version of 1964. Thus, according to the AFL-CIO's Andy Biemiller, "It is not utopian, but realistic, to say that, having waited so long, America can wait until the next Congress."[81]

The last plan to emerge in 1974—the Kennedy-Mills National Health Insurance Act—was something of an incremental compromise that incorporated aspects of all the major proposals. Mills and Kennedy were brought together at the behest of SSA Commissioner Bob Ball.[82] While Mills moved to the left after initially introducing Nixon's Comprehensive Health Insurance Act, Kennedy moved to the right after originally sponsoring organized labor's Health Security Act in 1971.[83]

Closely resembling Medicare, the Kennedy-Mills plan contained the financing features of labor's Health Security Act (a 4 percent increase in the Social Security payroll tax) along with Nixon's role for private insurers as fiscal intermediaries.[84] Kennedy-Mills also kept Medicare intact, unlike Nixon's and labor's plans that collapsed it into either a new, means-tested Federal Health Care Benefits scheme or a national Health Security program, respectively.[85] This decision did not garner the support of senior citizens' groups for Kennedy-Mills, but it did keep them from opposing the plan as they had others.[86]

With more and more politicians working toward a compromise plan, organized medicine became concerned that national health insurance might actually pass.[87] Wayne W. Bradley, then director of congressional relations for the AMA, remembered the Ways and Means' mark-up session as an extraordinary event: "There was an air of excitement, almost a feeling of destiny. After all, it was the first time that a major health insurance bill had come to a vote in committee since Medicare."[88] The AMA reintroduced a modified version of its 1971 Medicredit plan, which eventually garnered the most cosponsors (182), amounting to one-third of Congress. In contrast to its governing philosophy from the 1920s to the 1960s, the AMA's new conciliatory tone revealed how resigned it had become to the inevitability of dramatic change. The organization's new positions seemed to be in direct opposition to its previous ones: "In any program, we as physicians believe that the benefits should be comprehensive and uniform for all."[89] The AMA reinforced the perception of its willingness to compromise by publicly criticizing the country's methods of financing medical care: "The fact that our Medicredit bill now encompasses a catastrophic approach is testimony to the fact that we do indeed agree that there may be a fundamental mistake in how our country has approached insuring itself against the cost of illness."[90]

Labor's intransigence made efforts for compromise exceedingly difficult. Following President Nixon's resignation over Watergate on August 8, Chairman Mills attempted to forge another alternative. Following President Gerald Ford's exhortation on August 12 to pass a "good health bill," Mills moved to a centrist position by merging the Kennedy-Mills bill with Nixon's bill.[91] Despite Mills's political concessions, five conservative Southern Democrats on Ways and Means took note of labor's inflexibility and joined with seven Republicans in support of the AMA's Medicredit.[92] Thus, the final committee vote was only 13-12 in support of Mills's new compromise plan. "I've never tried harder on anything in my life than to bring about a consensus on this bill," said Mills. "But we don't have it. And I'm not going to the floor with a national health insurance bill approved by a 13-12 margin."[93]

In a great stroke of irony, one of the Democrats who refused to go along in support of Chairman Mills's proposal, Representative Sam Gibbons (Fla.), would eventually become chairman of Ways and Means in 1994. And he would lead the committee's drafting of a similar proposal to Mills's for radically expanding Medicare to achieve universal coverage, with the help of an employer mandate similar to that of President Nixon's plan: "A new public, self-financed insurance program, known as Medicare Part C," wrote Gibbons in 1994, "would be created as a safety net for those not served by private insurance."[94]

Desperate for some version of national health insurance, Representatives Martha Griffiths and James Corman (the original sponsors of labor's Health Security Act) suggested to Mills that he continue negotiating as they were now willing to compromise. "The President asked for a bill," Griffiths said. "I'm for giving him a bill."[95] Even President Ford himself indicated that he "still hoped Congress could approve a health insurance bill," which he labeled top priority legislation, before Congress adjourned.[96] This tactic failed, though, when labor absolutely refused to cooperate in any way.[97] "Essentially, we had worked out a proposal that Kennedy himself probably could have gone for and the administration, and Mills who at this point was seeing himself between the two," according to William Fullerton, one of the chief aides on the Ways and Means Committee and the individual Mills specifically charged with putting together a bill that would break the impasse on reform.[98] "We came close to that agreement but didn't make it. We didn't make it because of labor."[99] William Hsiao, Fullerton's colleague on the Ways and Means Committee staff who also helped

Mills in drafting his compromise national health insurance plan, largely concurs with Fullerton's assertion.[100]

Table 6.5
Brief Descriptions of the Four Major National Health Insurance Plans, 1974

Labor's Health Security	Kennedy-Mills's N.H.I.A.	Nixon's C.H.I.A.	AMA's Medicredit
The plan would provide comprehensive benefits for all Americans without deductibles or copayments. A new board within Health, Education, and Welfare would administer the program and the federal government would act as insurer. The program would be financed by federal general revenues and new payroll taxes of 1 percent of an employee's first $15,000 of income and 3.5 percent of an employer's entire payroll. Unearned income would be taxed at 1 percent.	The bill would require all employers and employees to participate in a new national program with standard benefits and provide the same coverage to the poor and Medicare participants. Employers would pay a new 3 percent and employees a new 1 percent payroll tax on the first $20,000 of income. Unearned income and federal welfare payments also would be taxed. An independent Social Security Administration would run the program and private insurers would act as financial intermediaries, but not pay claims. Each family would pay a maximum deductible of $300 before payments began and then pay 25 percent of all covered services. After a family with income above $8,800 had spent $1,000 out of its own pocket, the plan would provide catastrophic coverage. Maximum cost sharing for the poor would be related to income and a family of four with income under $4,800 would pay no deductibles or copayments.	The Nixon plan would require employers to offer insurance plans with standard benefits to their employees, but employee participation would be voluntary. After three years, employers would pay 75 percent of required premiums. The same benefits would be available to the poor in a new federal program and under Medicare. States would administer all but the Medicare program and private insurers would provide policies subject to state regulation. Employers and employees would pay premiums for their plans and the federal government would finance care of the poor and aged from general revenues and the Medicare Trust Fund. Each family would pay a maximum deductible of $450 before payments began and then 25 percent of all covered services. After a family had spent $1,500 out of its own pocket, the plan would cover all further "catastrophic" expenses. For families with income under $5,000, required deductibles and copayments would be related to income.	In a voluntary program, each family would receive a tax credit to cover premiums for standard plans. The credits would be given on a sliding scale depending on income, with the very poor receiving federal vouchers to cover premiums. The program would be administered by a federal advisory board and private insurers continue to provide all coverage. In effect, the plan would be financed by federal income tax revenues, with states financing a portion of coverage for the poor. Families would pay 20 percent of the first $500 for hospital care, first $500 of physician services and $500 of dental care. Catastrophic benefits would be provided after a family had spent 10 percent of its combined taxable income minus out-of-pocket expenses for basic benefits.

Source: "Brief Descriptions of 7 Major Health Insurance Programs Pending in Congressional Committees," *CQ Weekly Report* (July 20, 1974), 1862-63; Karen Davis, *National Health Insurance* (Washington, D.C.: The Brookings Institution, 1975), 166-71; and S. Davidson and T. Marmor, *The Cost of Living Longer* (Lexington, Mass.: Lexington Books, 1980), 97-106.

Following this stalemate in the Ways and Means Committee, Mills publicly lashed out at organized labor, saying that its "lack of support killed the Kennedy-Mills Bill."[101] In its editorial section, the *New York Times* agreed with Mills and others who accused labor of thwarting national health insurance: "Organized labor's 'all or nothing' position has been . . . directly responsible for scuttling an effective compromise."[102] Pure social security expansion for national health insurance had become blocked due Medicare's cost explosion.[103] Yet organized labor refused to support the incremental approach of Mills-Kennedy or to compromise to any alternative path of policymaking.[104] "Without labor's support, [attempts] at compromise had no chance," argues Starr. "Even though opposition to national health insurance had 'melted' away (as economist Alice Rivlin put it), none of the proposals could command a majority."[105]

Labor thought that compromise was not only unnecessary but also something to be positively avoided. Labor leaders were convinced that the 1974 mid-term elections would vindicate their rigid stance and that a "veto-proof" 94th Congress would be elected with many new, more liberal, members who would support the original Health Security Act.[106]

Organized Labor's Gamble Backfires

Labor turned to the mid-term elections in October 1974, hoping that Watergate would produce a wave of new, liberal Democrats, just as the elections of 1964 had done for Medicare.[108] Its political prediction proved accurate (table 6.6). The election ushered in seventy-five new representatives to the House, most of whom were Democrats and on record as supporting labor's plan.[108] Moreover, fifty-four congressmen who had cosponsored the AMA's Medicredit lost or retired.[109] The political environment suddenly appeared significantly more promising to labor and its fellow proponents of national health insurance.[110] Stunned by the magnitude of the Democrats' victory and the election's political implications, the AMA's president conceded that "his organization was willing to compromise"[111] from its voluntary plan—for the first time in its history—to one requiring that employers provide health insurance for their workers.[112]

Table 6.6
Party Composition of the House and Senate After Election Years, 1962-74

Congress	Year	House Democrats	House Republicans	Senate Democrats	Senate Republicans
88th	1962	258	176	68	32
89th	1964	295	140	67	33
90th	1966	248	187	64	36
91st	1968	243	192	58	42
92nd	1970	255	180	55	45
93rd	1972	243	192	57	43
94th	1974	290	145	61	39

Source: M. Kenneth Bowler, Robert Kudrle, and Theodore Marmor, "The Political Economy of National Health Insurance," in *Toward a National Health Policy*, ed. Warner, table 7-11.

But the demise of national health insurance occurred soon after the very mid-term elections that labor believed would lead to the unadulterated passage of its Health Security plan. First, Wilbur Mills's health and personal judgment had been deteriorating in 1974.[113] By late November, he and his committee faced assaults from many groups in Congress anxious for a greater role in policymaking.[114] On December 11, 1974, Mills withdrew as chairman of Ways and Means, citing his losing battle with alcoholism.[115] Power within his committee dispersed rapidly with a new chairman, twelve new, more liberal members,[116] and subcommittees in place by the end of December 1974.[117] In light of the country's deteriorating economy[118] and at the recommendation of his closest advisers,[119] Ford requested that no federal programs involving new spending be initiated.[120] His own ability to lead a struggle for national health insurance evaporated as his popularity ratings plummeted from a high of 71 percent (upon assuming office in August) to a low of 42 percent by December.[121]

The 94th Congress began 1975 with renewed efforts for universal coverage: "National health insurance will be one of the first bills—if not the first," House Speaker Carl Albert told the opening session of Congress.[122] Ways and Means Chairman Al Ullman seconded Speaker Albert's expectations: "Congress can no longer postpone major decisions to assure the availability of health services to all persons in the United States."[123] Ullman predicted passage of a plan by the summer of 1975.[124] Yet, in a interview with reporters prior to his 1975 State of the Union message, Ford reiterated his previous request that no federal programs involving new spending be initiated by threatening to veto them:

Question: Mr. President, your fiscal austerity program, because of that, will you have to abandon plans for national health insurance?

President Ford: Unfortunately, the "no new program guideline" that I laid down does mean the deferral of any recommendation by me of a national health insurance program, yes.[125]

With the new spending moratorium applied to national health insurance legislation, the Ford administration declined to reintroduce a proposal in 1975.[126] A slumping economy,[127] a growing national debt, mounting concerns over the long-term solvency of Social Security's OASDI trust funds,[128] and Ford's fiscal campaign to "whip inflation" closed one of national health insurance's most promising windows of opportunity.

Irreconcilable Differences: Social Security and Medicare's Divorce in 1977

The effort to pass national health insurance in 1974 represented one of the last gasps of Johnson's "Great Society" politics. According to Taylor Dark, the central pillars of this "order—a politically powerful labor movement, increasing economic growth and federal spending, and a working relationship between Democrats in Congress and the presidency"—were already unraveling with the arrival of economic "stagflation" and Jimmy Carter.[129] Redistributive politics gave way to regulatory politics, as attention shifted almost entirely from universal coverage to cost containment. As Starr observed: "The seemingly inexorable rise in entitlement programs gave Congress pause about any further additions to government responsibility. By fiscal year 1977, Medicare and Medicaid outlays were double what they had been only three years earlier. . . . Rising costs had driven health policy in the early seventies. Now, as one HEW official remarked, they were driving and paralyzing policy at the same time."[130]

In an effort to improve Medicare's operation, President Carter removed the program from the Social Security Administration's control in March 1977.[131] As Judith Feder explains: The "purpose was to unify administration of the federal government's two major health financing programs, Medicare and Medicaid, which had been run independently, and often without coordination, since their inception. Congress created a new agency, the Health Care Financing Administration (HCFA), to administer the programs."[132] According to President Jimmy Carter's HEW secretary, Joseph Califano, the primary reason for creating HCFA was to try to control costs through greater efficiency:

> *Califano*: I wanted to prove that the Great Society programs could be managed. That was number one. Number two, I wanted to get across to the liberals that you had to have competence and efficiency as well as compassion. There was no sense of efficiency among the liberal establishment, no sense of what that meant. . . .
>
> It was crazy to have Medicare and Medicaid separated. We lost all [bargaining] leverage [with doctors and hospitals]. And that's what it was about. The overall reorganization of HEW was to make it so I could run it, or anybody could run it. Sure, Carter wanted the government to be more efficient. That's one of the things he ran on. That's one of the things I admired about him. He understood the importance of that issue. Indeed, if we had more of that, we'd have less of what we have today in terms of the tremendous reaction to waste in the social programs.[133]

Removing Medicare from the SSA provided evidence that health insurance and old age benefits were structurally dissonant schemes. The SSA had designed and implemented Medicare "as a program for claims payments more than health care delivery."[134] But its ability to predict and at least marginally control OASDI's benefits did not carry over to Medicare, in part because benefits bore no relation to a beneficiary's contributions. The idea to remove Medicare from the SSA came from those who were deeply committed to social insurance.[135] Yet, many within the SSA were devastated: "The saddest day for Medicare is the day that Califano took the program away from Social Security and gave it to the Health Care Financing Administration. . . . Medicare was never the same after that."[136]

According to Theodore Marmor, however, "The creation of a comprehensive federal agency reflected the prediction that universal health insurance was to happen and the federal role in medical care finance should be consolidated."[137] Hale Champion, under secretary of HEW and Califano's top aide at the time, confirms Marmor's assertion that part of the motivation in creating HCFA was to advance the cause of national health insurance:

> *Edward Berkowitz*: You hinted before that the objective was in part to bring this new relationship to the medical programs and create a national basis for national health insurance, but in the end Medicare and Medicaid remained separate. We never got national health insurance. We still don't have national health insurance, and what we got instead was a separate agency.
>
> *Champion*: Yes.
>
> *Berkowitz*: Was that a fair characterization?
>
> *Champion*: Well, yes.[138]

As Marmor has observed, that was neither the first nor the last time that the conceptions of Medicare adjustments were dominated by ambitious notions of what the larger role of federal health policy should be. Following HCFA's creation, President Carter did broach the issue of national health insurance, particularly in connection to his renomination struggle with Senator Edward Kennedy in late 1979 and early 1980.[139] Organized labor even came to embrace employer mandates and retaining a major role for commercial insurers, despite its earlier unbending insistence on pure, Social Security-styled national health insurance.[140] But neither Carter's nor labor's efforts led to any serious congressional consideration and the 1970s ended as the decade, in the words of Mark Peterson, "when the hopes and opportunities for revamping health care financing were at their 20th-century zenith."[141]

Conclusion

With policymakers' flawed design, Medicare became such an expensive entitlement that it ceased to be an add-on to Social Security and evolved into a separate program in its own right and with its own administrator, the Health Care Financing Administration. The success policymakers enjoyed in adding protection to Social Security came at a programmatic cost. Medicare's structure and subsequent profligacy led to a system that eventually priced itself out of contention for any expansion that could cover the 10 percent of the population, or 23 million individuals, without health insurance.

Interest group activity played a critical role in producing a legislative stalemate over the issue of national health insurance in 1974. Ironically, organized labor's insistence on adhering to its plan for pure social insurance scuttled any chance for political compromise at the time when compromise appeared more imminent than ever before. The public path of pure social insurance expansion, as represented by labor's Health Security Act, was clearly blocked. But organized labor lobbied successfully to prevent an exit to any new path of policymaking (such as Nixon's employer mandates). In the process, labor's position also blocked the other—arguably more incremental—alternative of Kennedy-Mills, which most closely resembled a major expansion of Medicare.

Under more ordinary political and economic circumstances, labor's opposition alone would probably not have been capable of blocking reform. But in the context of both Watergate and a rapidly deteriorating economy that had already been experiencing severe inflation problems, the margin for disagreement was significantly narrowed. And the margin was narrow despite the fact that Watergate may very well have made national health insurance more possible in the first place. Why? Because the "Nixon administration was eager to enact a popular program," notes Wainess, "that could deflect attention away from the scandal."[142] Nevertheless, every interest group had to compromise for anything substantial to pass.

Even if labor had come out in support of some form of compromise, it is still far from certain that a national health insurance plan of any kind would have passed in Congress. But what is clear is that labor's unbending opposition made a difficult political situation completely intractable. After this golden opportunity for change passed, the federal government would be consumed in the following decades with trying to control the costs of Medicare and OASDI.

Notes

1. See Jaap Kooijman, . . . *And the Pursuit of National Health: The Incremental Strategy toward National Health Insurance* (Amsterdam: Rodopi, 1999).

2. Robert Ball, "Medicare's Roots: What Medicare's Architects Had in Mind," *Generations* 20 (Summer 1996): 13.

3. See Board of Trustees of the Federal Hospital Insurance Trust Fund, *1971 Annual Report of the Board of Trustees of the Federal Hospital Insurance Trust Fund*, 92nd Congress, 1st Session, House Document No. 92-87 (1971); Board of Trustees of Federal Supplementary Insurance Trust Fund, *1971 Annual Report of the Board of Trustees of the Federal Supplementary Insurance Trust Fund*, 92nd Congress, 1st Session, House Document No. 92-89 (1971); and "Social Security and Welfare Proposals," *Hearing before the House Committee on Ways and Means*, 91st Congress, 1st Session (October 15-November 13, 1969), 187-97.

4. On "M Day" (July 1, 1966), a 19-million-person demographic group, the nation's retirees, instantaneously had health insurance coverage. They had contributed next to nothing for their Medicare coverage during their years of employment, making the program a costly pay-as-you-go scheme from the beginning.

5. Judith Feder, *Medicare: The Politics of Federal Hospital Insurance* (Lexington, Mass.: Lexington Books, 1977), vii.

6. "National Health Insurance: A Concept Whose Time Has Come," *Journal of Accountancy* 138 (July 1974): 25; "National Health Insurance Is on the Way," *Business Week*, January 26, 1974, 70; "NHI: Here Comes the Main Event," *Medical World News* 15 (March 1, 1974): 15.

7. "Nixon's Health Insurance Plan Going to the Hill," *Washington Post*, January 19, 1974, A1.

8. "Nixon Sees Passage in '74 of Health Insurance Plan," *New York Times*, February 6, 1974, 16.

9. *1973 Annual Report of the Board of Trustees of the Federal Old-Age and Survivors Insurance and Disability Insurance Trust Funds* (Washington, D.C.: GPO, 1974), 31; "Social Security: Promising Too Much to Too Many?" *U.S. News & World Report*, July 15, 1974, 26-30; "A Long Look at the SSS," *Wall Street Journal*, July 15, 1974, 10; and "No Kidding, Mr. Meany," *Wall Street Journal*, August 23, 1974, 6.

10. Joseph A. Califano Jr., *Governing America* (New York: Simon & Schuster, 1981), 102. See also, "Round Table: The Future of the Social Security System," *Financing Social Security*, ed. Colin Campbell (Washington, D.C.: American Enterprise Institute, 1979), 350.

11. *Wall Street Journal*, December 9, 1977, 1; and "National Health Insurance," *1979 CQ Almanac* (Washington, D.C.: CQ Press, 1980), 537: "Ways and Means Chairman Al Ullman was unsympathetic to more payroll taxes."

12. Gaston Rimlinger in *Social Security: The First Half-Century*, ed. G. Nash, N. Pugach, and R. Tomasson (Albuquerque: University of New Mexico Press, 1988), 110.

13. Paul Samuelson, "On Social Security," *Newsweek,* February 13, 1967, 88.

14. See Jerry L. Mashaw, *The Bureaucratic State* (New Haven, Conn.: Yale University Press, 1983); and Deborah Stone, *The Disabled State* (Philadelphia: Temple University Press, 1984).

15. Cohen, "From Medicare to National Health Insurance," in *Toward a New Human* Rights, ed. David C. Warner (Austin, Tex.: Lyndon Baines Johnson School of Public Affairs, 1977), 151.

16. Samuelson, "On Social Security," 88: "The beauty about social insurance is that it is actuarially unsound. Everyone who reaches retirement age is given benefit privileges that far exceed his payments by more than ten times as much (or five times, counting in employer payments)!

How is this possible? It stems from the fact that the national product is growing at compound interest and can be expected to do so as far ahead as the eye cannot see. Always there are more youths than old folks in a growing population. More important, with real incomes growing at some 3 per cent per year, the taxable base upon which benefits rest in any period are (sic) much greater than the taxes paid historically by the generation now retired. And social security, unlike actuarially funded insurance, is untouched by inflation" (italics in original).

For more on this assumption by policymakers, see Irwin Wolkstein, "Medicare's Financial Status—How Did We Get There?" in *Conference on the Future of Medicare*, Committee on Ways and Means, U.S. House of Representatives, 98th Congress, 1st Session (November 29, 1983), 16: "The time of Medicare's enactment was also a period of optimism in thinking about the future of the Nation's economy. Continuing high rates of economic growth were generally expected."

17. *1973 Annual Report of the Board of Trustees of the Federal Old-Age Insurance and Survivors Insurance and Disability Trust Funds* (Washington, D.C.: GPO, 1974), 31; "Social Security: Promising Too Much to Too Many?" *U.S. News & World Report*, July 15, 1974, 26-30; and "A Long Look at the SSS," *Wall Street Journal*, July 15, 1974, editorial, 10, and "No Kidding, Mr. Meany," August 23, 1974, editorial, 6.

18. See "Medicare and Medicaid: Problems, Issues, and Alternatives," *Report of the Staff to the Committee on Finance*, U.S. Senate (Washington, D.C.: GPO, 1970).

19. For complete account of Medicare's daunting implementation, see Herman A. Somers and Anne R. Somers, *Medicare and the Hospitals: Issues and Prospects* (Wash-

ington, D.C.: The Brookings Institution, 1967); and Feder, *Medicare: The Politics of Federal Hospital Insurance*.

20. Theodore Marmor, *The Politics of Medicare*, 2d ed. (New York: Aldine de Gruyter, 2000), 96-99.

21. Lawrence D. Brown, "Technocratic Corporatism and Administrative Reform in Medicare," *Journal of Health Politics, Policy and Law* 10 (1985): 581-83.

22. Philip Booth, ed., *Social Security: Policy for the Seventies, Proceedings of the Seventh Social Security Conference* (Ann Arbor, Mich.: Institute of Labor and Industrial Relations, 1973), 72-73, italics added. Herman Somers corroborated this conclusion from his own first hand account of Medicare's implementation: "Not surprisingly, the final product was different from any of the early proposals. Equally unsurprising, Medicare proved no exception to the rule that the legislative process rarely produces large or sudden upheavals, that it rarely imposes programs out of context with the existing social and economic environment. Almost inescapably, for good or ill, Medicare was adapted to existing medical care and financing practices and institutions" (Somers and Somers, *Medicare and the Hospitals*, 17)."

23. Cohen, "From Medicare to National Health Insurance," 146-47.

24. Marmor, *The Politics of Medicare*, 2d ed., 99.

25. Cohen to the Secretary, and Cohen to the President, March 8, 1967, both Box 91, Cohen Papers, as cited in E. Berkowitz, "The Historical Development of Social Security in the United States," in *Social Security in the 21st Century*, ed. E. Kingson and J. Schulz (New York: Oxford University Press, 1997), 36.

26. "Congress Lags on Health Insurance," *New York Times*, May 27, 1974, 52.

27. "Medicare: A Fifteen-Year Perspective," *Hearings before the Select Committee on Aging, House of Representatives*, 96th Congress, 2nd Session (July 30, 1980), Comm. Pub. No. 96-258, 14: "We didn't fund it properly to begin with; that is part A. We've had some troubles with Part A ever since the first funding. We started off with I believe 0.5 funding, combined tax on employer-employee. It should have been about 0.9. Within 3 years we found the costs had risen much faster than we had anticipated. So, we were in trouble then and we remained in trouble for some time with the fund, and I assume that we are still in trouble of financing it."

For more on Medicare and Medicaid's financial problems, see "History of the Rising Costs of the Medicare and Medicaid Programs and Attempts to Control These Costs: 1966-1975," Department of Health, Education, and Welfare (Washington, D.C.: U.S. General Accounting Office, 1976).

28. Marmor, *The Politics of Medicare*, 2d ed., 96-99; Paul Starr, *The Social Transformation of American Medicine* (New York: Basic Books, 1982), 374-76.

29. Marmor, *The Politics of Medicare*, 374-76.

30. Judith M. Feder, "The Social Security Administration and Medicare: A Strategy of Implementation," in *Toward a National Health Policy: Public Policy and the Control of Health-Care Costs*, ed. Kenneth Friedman and Stuart Rakoff (Lexington, Mass.: Lexington Books, 1977), 19. See also, Feder, *Medicare: The Politics of Federal Hospital Insurance*, 149; and "Recollections (Discussions) by Social Security Administration Officials' Knowledge and/or Involvement in Certain Stages of Early Implementation of the Medicare Program" (Calendar Year 1966), SSA Regional Office, Atlanta (September 25, 1992), 18-19, provided to the author by Mr. Arthur Hess.

31. Starr, *The Social Transformation of American Medicine*, 385.

32. Howard West, "Five Years of Medicare--A Statistical Review," *Social Security Bulletin* 34 (December 1971): 21.

33. Rosemary Stevens, *In Sickness and in Wealth: American Hospitals in the Twentieth Century* (New York: Basic Books, 1989), 284.

34. "The Rapid Rise of Hospital Costs," Executive Office of the President's Council on Wage and Price Stability Staff Report (Washington, D.C.: GPO, January 1977), 9-11.

35. For more information on these dynamics, see Martin Feldstein, *Hospital Costs and Health Insurance* (Cambridge, Mass.: Harvard University Press, 1981), 176, 306. See also, "Expenditures for Health Care: Federal Programs and Their Effects," Congressional Budget Office (Washington, D.C.: GPO, 1977), 5; and Feder, *Medicare: The Politics of Federal Hospital Insurance*, 143: "The Medicare law promised to pay for medical care for the elderly without interfering in its delivery. But this promise ignored a basic economic fact: How care is paid for significantly influences the quantity and quality of care delivered. Thus a payment program necessarily interferes in the practice of medicine. If an agreement to pay for care has no strings attached, it removes any fiscal constraints on physicians' and hospitals' development and delivery of medical services."

36. See Staff Report, "Medicare and Medicaid: Problems, Issues, and Alternatives," *Senate Committee on Finance*, 91st Congress, 1st Session (February 1970), 4.

37. "Summary of Major Provisions of P.L. 89-97, the Social Security Amendments of 1965," *House Committee on Ways and Means*, House of Representatives, 89th Congress, 1st Session (September 1965), part F "Statistical Data," 20-21. See also, "Administration of Medicare Cost-Saving Experiments," *Hearings before the Subcommittee on Oversight, Committee on Ways and Means*, House of Representatives, 94th Congress, 2nd Session (May 14-17, 1976); and "History of the Rising Costs of the Medicare and Medicaid Programs and Attempts to Control These Costs, 1966-1975," Department of Health, Education, and Welfare (Washington, D.C.: GPO, 1976).

38. "Summary of Major Provisions of P.L. 89-97." See also, *The Budget of the United States Government*, Executive Office of the President, Fiscal Year 1981 (Washington, D.C.: GPO), 245; and Senate Report 89-404, 85, n1.

39. Marmor, *The Politics of Medicare*, 2d ed., 98-99.

40. Stevens, *In Sickness and in Wealth*, 284-93.

41. M. Gornick, et. al., "Thirty Years of Medicare: Impact on the Covered Population," in U.S. Department of Health and Human Services, *Health Care Financing Review*, "Medicare: Advancing Towards the 21st Century 1966-96," 184.

42. Jonathan Oberlander, "Medicare and the American State: The Politics of Federal Health Insurance, 1965-1995" (Ph.D. dissertation, Yale University, 1995), 219-43.

43. The monthly premiums of participating senior citizens contributed only 50 percent of Part B's total costs. Moreover, the elderly's share of Part B's costs dropped to 25 percent by 1983, because the increase in their premium rate was limited to the percent increase in OASI benefits, which rose much slower than increases in medical costs.

44. "The Reform of Health Care Systems: Review of Seventeen OECD Countries," Organization for Economic Cooperation and Development (Paris: OECD, 1994) 37.

45. Oberlander, "Medicare and the American State," 229.

46. Jacob Javits, *Javits: The Autobiography of a Public Man* (Boston: Houghton Mifflin, 1981), 301.

47. Flint J. Wainess, "The Ways and Means of National Health Care Reform, 1974 and Beyond," *Journal of Health Politics, Policy and Law* 24 (April 1999): 308. Wainess's comprehensive account of the national health insurance debate in 1974 is one of the very few on this seminal period of political history.

48. Godfrey Hodgson, "The Politics of American Health Care," *Atlantic Monthly*, October 1973.

49. "Nixon's Health Insurance Plan Going to Hill," *Washington Post*, January 19, 1974, A1.

50. *New York Times*, February 2, 1974, editorial, 28.

51. *Washington Post*, May 26, 1974, editorial, C6.

52. "Insuring the National Health," *Newsweek*, June 3, 1974, 73.

53. *New York Times Magazine*, July 21, 1974, 10: "That some form of national health insurance will be enacted . . . seems virtually certain. In the years between Truman and Nixon, the argument has shifted from 'whether' to 'what kind.' Even organized medicine no longer quivers at the thought."

54. "Health Insurance Package Unveiled by Wilbur Mills," *Washington Post*, August 15, 1974, 1.

55. Title of Wilbur Cohen's chapter in *Toward New Human Rights: The Social Policies of the Kennedy and Johnson Administrations*, ed. David Warner (Austin, Tex.: Lyndon B. Johnson School of Public Affairs, 1977), 143-55.

56. See Marie Gottschalk, *The Shadow Welfare State: Labor, Business, and the Politics of Health Care in the United States* (Ithaca, N.Y.: Cornell University Press, 2000), 68-74.

57. "Health Care Now: On a Cold Day in 1971, President Richard M. Nixon's Speech to Congress, February 18, 1971," *New Republic*, September 19, 1994, 11.

58. Private insurance carriers were attracted to the requirement in Nixon's plan that employers purchase private insurance. They were concerned, however, that many of the new beneficiaries from this mandate would be those who required lots of medical care and, thus, be unprofitable.

59. For more information on labor's position, see "Statement by the AFL-CIO Executive Council on National Health Insurance," Bal Harbour, Florida (February 20, 1967).

60. "The Case for National Health Insurance," *AFL-CIO American Federationist*, January 1970, 9-10.

61. "National Health Insurance Proposals," *Hearings before the Committee on Ways and Means, House of Representatives*, 92nd Congress, 1st session (October 19 and 20, 1971), 287-89. See also, "Woodcock Asks for Health Plan Modeled on Social Security," *New York Times*, October 29, 1971, 23.

62. David C. Jacobs, "The UAW and the Committee for National Health Insurance," *Advances in Industrial and Labor Relations*, vol. 4 (Greenwich, Conn.: JAI Press, 1987), 126.

63. "National Health Security: A Clear Answer," *AFL-CIO American Federationist*, June 1971, 6.

64. "The Right to Health Care," *AFL-CIO American Federationist*, September 1972, 14.

65. "National Health Insurance Proposals," *Hearings before Committee on Ways and Means*, 593.

66. See Lawrence D. Brown, *Politics and Health Care Organization: HMO's as Federal Policy* (Washington, D.C.: The Brookings Institution, 1983); and Starr, *The Social Transformation of American Medicine*, 396.

67. See Joseph P. Newhouse, Charles E. Phelps, and William B. Schwartz, *Policy Options and the Impact of National Health Insurance* (Santa Monica, Calif.: Rand, June 1974); *National Health Insurance Proposals* (Washington, D.C.: AEI Press, November 13, 1974); Allen D. Spiegel and Simon Podair, *Medicaid: Lessons for National Health Insurance* (Rockville, Md.: Aspen Systems Corporation, 1975).

68. "Health Insurance: Prospects for Passage Dim," *CQ Weekly Report*, July 20, 1974, 1861.

69. See "Insuring the Nation's Health," *Newsweek*, June 3, 1974; John K. Inglehart, "National Health Insurance Tops Ways and Means Agenda," *National Journal of Reports* 6 (March 16, 1974): 383; and Alice Rivlin, "Agreed: Here Comes National Health Insurance," *New York Times Magazine*, July 21, 1974.

70. "Insuring the Nation's Health," Inglehart, "National Health Insurance Tops Ways and Means Agenda," and Rivlin, "Agreed: Here Comes National Health Insurance."

71. See Allen J. Matusow, *Nixon's Economy: Booms, Busts, Dollars, and Votes* (Lawrence: University Press of Kansas, 1998), 287-88.

72. See Saul Waldman, *National Health Insurance Proposals: Provisions of Bills Introduced in the 93rd Congress as of October 1973* (Washington, D.C.: Department of HEW), Social Security Administration, Office of Research and Statistics.

73. "Health Bill: One More Try," *Washington Post*, August 6, 1974, A11.

74. "Brief Descriptions of 7 Major Health Insurance Programs Considered in 1974," *1974 CQ Almanac* (Washington, D.C.: GPO, 1975), 388-89.

75. "Kennedy Losing Some Support on Health Aid Bill," *Washington Post*, April 17, 1974, A20.

76. "Labor Hardens Opposition to Compromise Health Bill," *Washington Post*, April 30, 1974, A2.

77. "Labor Hardens Opposition to Compromise Health Bill," and "Labor Refuses Compromised Insurance Bill," *Washington Post*, May 18, 1974, A13.

78. "National Health Insurance," *Hearings before the Committee on Ways and Means, House of Representatives*, 93rd Congress, 2nd Session, vol. 3 (May 3, 10, and 17, 1974), 1421-23.

79. "The Health Insurance Debate," *Washington Post*, May 26, 1974, editorial, C6: "If a workable compromise is to be effected, one more voice must be raised in its favor: the voice of organized labor, which, for good reasons, carries weight on Capitol Hill in discussions of health insurance. So far the major unions have rejected all three bills. They are holding out for a far more drastic 'health security' bill that would replace all existing health insurance, public and private, with a single federally-run system and would provide free care for everyone. . . . Even the AMA is no longer opposing national health insurance as such."

80. "Letters to the Editor: Labor's Case for Health Legislation," *Washington Post*, July 5, 1974, A17. See also "National Health Insurance: Diagnosing the Alternatives," *AFL-CIO American Federationist*, June 1974, 7: "In April 1974, Sen. Edward M. Kennedy (D-Mass.), who had been a principal sponsor of Health Security, and Rep. Wilbur Mills (D-Ark.), introduced what they called a 'compromise' bill. While on balance Mills-Kennedy is an improvement over the Nixon bill, it falls far short of meeting the need. The AFL-CIO's conclusion that only National Health Security meets the needs of all Americans becomes clearer when the Nixon bill and the Mills-Kennedy bill are contrasted with the Health Security."

81. "Letters to the Editor: Labor's Case for Health Legislation," *Washington Post*, July 5, 1974, A17. See also "National Health Insurance: Diagnosing the Alternatives," *AFL-CIO American Federationist*, June 1974, 7.

82. Edward Berkowitz, HCFA Oral History Interview with William Fullerton (Washington, D.C., 1995), 10.

83. For a wealth of background material on maneuvers on the House of Representative's side, particularly the Ways and Means Committee, see *National Health*

Insurance Resource Book, prepared by the Staff of the Committee on Ways and Mean for the Use of the Committee (Washington, D.C.: GPO, April 11, 1974).

84. See Wainess, "The Ways and Means of National Health Care Reform, 1974 and Beyond," 318-19.

85. *National Health Insurance Proposals*, 47-51.

86. "Nixon Presses Health Plan: Would Accept Compromise," *Washington Post*, May 21, 1974, A4.

87. Frank Campion, *The AMA and U.S. Health Policy since 1940* (Chicago: Chicago Review Press, 1984), 320-24.

88. Campion, *The AMA and U.S. Health Policy Since 1940*, 322.

89. "National Health Insurance," *Hearings before the Committee on Ways and Means, House of Representatives*, 93rd Congress, 2nd Session, vol. 2 (April 24, 25, and 26, 1974), 806.

90. "National Health Insurance," 820.

91. "Mills Panel Drafts New Plan," *Washington Post*, August 20, 1974, p. A1; "Parts of Health-Care Bill are Approved by Mills Panel in Tentative, Close Votes," *Wall Street Journal*, August 21, 1974, 4.

92. "Health Insurance: Committee Bogs Down," *CQ Weekly Report*, August 24, 1974, 2275: Democrats—Landrum (Ga.), Fulton (Tenn.), Burleson (Tex.), Gibbons (Fla.), and Waggonner (La.).

93. "Health Insurance: Committee Bogs Down." See also, Campion, *The AMA and U.S. Health Policy since 1940*, 323.

94. The Honorable Sam M. Gibbons, acting chairman, Committee on Ways and Means, "The Chairman's Health Care Reform Mark, Summary" (Washington, D.C.: June 6, 1994), 1.

95. "Health Insurance: No Action in 1974," *1974 CQ Almanac*, 391-94.

96. "National Health Insurance," *CQ Weekly Report*, August 31, 1974, 2345.

97. "A Health Bill That Wasn't and Why," *Medical World News*, September 13, 1974, 17: "When Mills reached agreement with Senator Edward Kennedy on a compromise bill, Kennedy's major national health insurance backer—organized labor—balked and insisted on its own bill, the draft Health Security Act, or nothing."

98. Wainess, "The Ways and Means of National Health Care Reform, 1974 and Beyond," 324.

99. Edward Berkowitz, HCFA Oral History Interview with William Fullerton (Washington, D.C., 1995), 11.

100. Edward Berkowitz, HCFA Oral History Interview with William Hsiao (Cambridge, Mass., August 23, 1995), 4.

101. "Health Bill Seen Dead This Year," *Washington Post*, August 22, 1974, A1.

102. "Walkout on Health," *New York Times*, August 23, 1974, editorial, 28: "The abrupt decision by committee chairman Wilbur D. Mills, co-sponsor of that eminently sensible proposal, to shelve efforts to enact a health insurance bill because 'there is no majority consensus now' represents an irresponsible surrender to . . . special interest lobbies—one supporting unrealistically utopian insurance plans."

103. Richard Lyons, "U.S. Health Insurance: A Legislative Goal That Has No Foes Stalled by Differences in Approach," *New York Times*, August 27, 1974, 20: "When organized labor started a push for enactment of national health insurance in 1969, Mr. Mills was wary. He felt that he had been burned badly and perhaps even lied to, by members of the Johnson Administration, on the finances of Medicare, which had swollen enormously in cost. The Johnson Administration had, in effect, traded off meaningful cost controls in

Medicare in order to get the votes to enact the program. Mr. Mills has said repeatedly that he is not going to get burned again."

104. Wainess, "The Ways and Means of National Health Care Reform, 1974 and Beyond," 330.

105. Starr, *Social Transformation of American Medicine*, 405.

106. "Labor Hold-Out," *1974 CQ Almanac*, 387.

107. "Labor Hold-Out," *1974 CQ* Almanac, 387.

108. Gottschalk, *The Shadow Welfare State*, 74.

109. "Health Insurance: No Action in 1974," *1974 CQ Almanac*, 394.

110. "Labor Flexes Its Legislative Muscle," *Nation's Business*, January 1975, 58: "Probably the most prized legislative goal of big labor this year is passage of a national health insurance bill, and it will exert maximum pressure on Congress to go with the original version proposed to the 93rd Congress by Senator Kennedy and Representative Griffiths."

111. "AMA Open to Compromise on a Plan for Health Insurance," *New York Times*, October 8, 1974.

112. "National Health Insurance," *1975 CQ Almanac* (Washington, D.C.: GPO, 1976), 636.

113. Julian Zelizer, *Taxing America: Wilbur D. Mills, Congress, and the State, 1945-1975* (Cambridge: Cambridge University Press, 1998), 350-53.

114. "Weakened Mills and His Committee Face Rough Going," *Wall Street Journal*, 29 November 29, 1974, 1.

115. "Ways and Means Panel with Mills Gone," *Wall Street Journal*, December 11, 1974, 4.

116. "Mills Quits as Chairman; Young Democrats Advance," *New York Times*, December 11, 1974, 1.

117. See Randall Strahan, *New Ways and Means: Reform and Change in a Congressional Committee* (Chapel Hill, N.C.: University of North Carolina Press, 1990).

118. "Congress is Urged to Act on Economy," *Washington Post*, December 3, 1974, A1; "The Economy: A Crisis of Confidence," *Washington Post*, December 11, 1974, editorial, A19; "Ford: 'All of Us Must Renew and Invigorate Our Economy,'" *Washington Post*, December 12, 1974, A8; "Economic Signs Worsen as Auto Layoffs Rise," *Washington Post*, December 19, 1974, A1; "The Economy: Time is Growing Short," *Washington Post*, December 19, 1974, editorial, A15; and "Recession or Depression and How Deep?" *New York Times*, December 25, 1974, editorial, 33.

119. Personal interview with President Gerald Ford's secretary of HEW, Caspar Weinberger (September 5, 1998). See also, "Ford Gets Options to Improve Economy," *New York Times*, 22 December 22, 1974, 27.

120. "Ford Signs Antitrust Bill; 2 Vetoes Attack Spending," *New York Times*, December 24, 1974, 1.

121. "Ford Rating in Poll Slips to Low of 42%," *New York Times*, December 26, 1974, 1.

122. "National Health Insurance," *1975 CQ Almanac* (Washington, D.C.: GPO, 1976), 636.

123. "National Health Insurance," *1975 CQ Almanac*, 636.

124. "National Health Insurance," *1975 CQ* Almanac, 636.

125. Congressional Quarterly, "Texts of Ford News Conferences," in *Presidency 1975* (Washington, D.C.: CQ Press, 1976), 45-A, 46-A.

126. "National Health Insurance," *1975 CQ Almanac*, 636.

127. Matusow, *Nixon's Economy*, 300-302.

128. *1973 Annual Report of the Board of Trustees of the Federal Old-Age and Survivors Insurance and Disability Insurance Trust Funds* (Washington, D.C.: GPO, 1974), 31; "Social Security: Promising Too Much to Too Many?" *U.S. News & World Report*, July 15, 1974, 26-30; "A Long Look at the SSS," *Wall Street Journal*, July 15, 1974, 10; and "No Kidding, Mr. Meany," *Wall Street Journal*, August 23, 1974, 6.

129. Taylor Dark, "Organized Labor and the Carter Administration," in *The Presidency and Domestic Politics of Jimmy Carter*, ed. Howard Rosenbaum and A. Ugrinsky (Westport, Conn.: Greenwood Press, 1994), 779. See also, Steve Fraser and Gary Gerstle, eds., *The Rise and Fall of the New Deal Order, 1930-1980* (Princeton, N.J.: Princeton University Press, 1989).

130. Starr, *The Social Transformation of American Medicine*, 406. See also, John Inglehart, "The Rising Costs of Health Care—Something Must be Done, but What?" *National Journal*, October 16, 1976.

131. For an interesting perspective on HCFA's creation and evolution, see Edward Berkowitz, HCFA Oral History Interview with Jay Constantine (Alexandria, Va., August 24, 1995).

132. Feder, *Medicare: The Politics of Federal Hospital Insurance*, vii.

133. Edward Berkowitz, HCFA Oral History Interview with Joseph Califano (New York City, August 31, 1995), 1-2.

134. Feder, *Medicare: The Politics of Federal Hospital Insurance*, 154.

135. J. W. Van Gorkom, *Social Security Revisited* (Washington, D.C.: American Enterprise Institute, 1977), 32: "Without in any way criticizing the function and merits of Medicare, I think it should not be combined with OASDI benefits, [because] Medicare is not an income maintenance program nor are its benefits in any way related to earnings. . . It is combined with the OASDI program only through expediency and administrative convenience." See also, Report of the 1979 Advisory Council on Social Security, U.S. House of Representatives (Washington, D.C.: GPO, 1980), ix.

136. "Recollections by Social Security Administration Officials' Knowledge and/or Involvement in Certain Stages of Early Implementation of the Medicare Program," 20.

137. Marmor, *The Politics of Medicare*, 2d ed., 118, 156.

138. Edward Berkowitz, HCFA Oral History Interview with Hale Champion (Cambridge, Mass., August 9, 1995), 11.

139. See Robert Finbow, "Presidential Leadership or Structural Constraints? The Failure of President Carter's Health Insurance Proposals," *Presidential Studies Quarterly* 28 (Winter 1998): 169-87; Martin Halpern, "Jimmy Carter and the UAW: Failure of an Alliance," *Presidential Studies Quarterly* 26 (Summer 1996): 755-77; and Starr, *Social Transformation of American Medicine*, 412-14.

140. Gottschalk, *The Shadow Welfare State*, 78-85.

141. Mark Peterson, "Institutional Change and the Health Politics of the 1990s," *American Behavioral Scientist* 36 (July-August 1996): 782.

142. Wainess, "The Ways and Means of National Health Care Reform, 1974 and Beyond," 307.

CHAPTER SEVEN

Locked In and Crowded Out

Entrenched Paths and Accumulated Costs
Impede Universal Coverage
(1980s and 1990s)

Bringing health insurance within the reach of every American family was the final piece of the Social Security system the Democrats had begun assembling under Franklin Roosevelt. It represented the single most important unfulfilled commitment of that party to its working-class and middle-class base.

—**Donna Shalala**
President Clinton's Secretary of Health and Human Services (1993)

Universal coverage did not become a high-profile public issue again until the early 1990s. Prior to this, the country's most expensive entitlement programs, Medicare and Social Security's OASDI, ran into severe financial difficulty, which forced the government to experiment with ways to control costs. Without successful cost control, expanded health insurance coverage could not be feasible. Nonetheless, the recession in 1991 propelled the issue of universal coverage back onto the public agenda, and its prominence continued to rise during the presidential campaign of 1992.

Unfortunately, the accumulated costs of OASDI and Medicare—together with the decades of policymaking that produced them—locked policymakers into a perverse situation. On the one hand, policymakers could not expand either program, because their massive financial obligations had exhausted their means of financing: the payroll tax. The high costs of Medicare and OASDI effectively crowded out any additional program coverage or development financed by the payroll tax. But, on the other hand, lock-in effects from years of policymaking, which had created the two programs' vast commitments, blocked any exit to a new path. This fragmented health care system (with employer-provided and tax-

109

subsidized insurance for workers, Medicare for senior citizens, Medicaid for the poor, the Veterans' Administration for veterans) made comprehensive change for the purposes of achieving universal coverage a threatening and irreconcilable proposition for the many organizations and individuals with a stake in the system as it existed.

Lock-in effects are another way of saying that major policy initiatives have major social consequences. "Individuals make important commitments in response to certain types of government action," as Paul Pierson observes, and these commitments, in turn, "vastly increase the disruption by new policies, effectively locking in previous decisions."[1] President Clinton's dramatic attempt at comprehensive health care reform in 1993-94 graphically illustrated the futility of trying to reconcile old institutional arrangements with new policy paths. The costs of inherited programs and the numerous political constituencies that developed in strong support of them blocked any exit to a new and comprehensive path of universal coverage.

Ultimately, the private path of tax-subsidized, employer-provided health insurance and the public path of separate government programs for specific segments of the population constitute the nation's medical-industrial complex. This complex, with its fragmented configuration of political agents and interests loyal to their public programs or private arrangements, effectively resists the rare attempts by policymakers to exit to a new path for the purposes of universal coverage.

System Rationalization in the 1980s: Cost-Control Imperative

Out of financial necessity, Congress made an epochal change to Medicare in 1983. It switched the program to a prospective payment system (PPS), a pre-designated method of hospital reimbursement.[2] The change proved effective in slowing Medicare's rate of cost increase. But as an unintended consequence, much of the program's cost reduction came at the expense of hospitals' cost-shifting from public to private patients.

Cost-shifting dramatically induced the growth of managed care in the latter 1980s, as employers sought to restrain the annual increases in their health insurance premiums. The problem of escalating private insurance premiums was not new, but cost-shifting exacerbated it and led to unprecedented annual increases of between 20 and 40 percent following the implementation of Medicare's new PPS.[3] Therefore, prepaid comprehensive health coverage—provided, for example, by HMOs—became not only attractive but also necessary for small to mid-sized companies that could neither afford to self-insure nor negotiate sufficient bargains with corporate carriers.

Prospective payment succeeded in switching the balance of political power from medical providers to the government. Yet, Medicare reform and the private sector's subsequent rationalization rendered universal coverage harder to attain. Why? Because reform and rationalization addressed serious problems associated with both Medicare and the private insurance industry, not the uninsured. As a result, the vast majority of Americans continued to possess adequate coverage against the cost of illness. The only difference was that the annual rate of increase in health care costs and insurance slowed. This trend decreased the saliency of the uninsured, because most people had some form of health insurance protection. It would take a recession in the early 1990s and a new surge of medical inflation to resurrect the issue of comprehensive reform.

How Medicare Reform Inadvertently Triggered the Rise of Managed Care

The conventional wisdom on how managed care came to replace traditional fee-for-service reimbursement as the nation's dominant mode of health insurance is that enlightened businesses and employers led the way in responding to the emergence of market forces in health care in the 1980s.[4] A common textbook treatment of managed care's ascendancy puts it this way: "Transformation of the health care delivery system through managed care [was] driven principally by market forces, and reinforced by government."[5] The irony is that the reverse is a more accurate portrayal of what happened. As this chapter endeavors to demonstrate, the transformation of the health care system through managed care was driven principally—albeit indirectly—by government, and then reinforced by market forces. In other words, before business behavior was a cause of managed care's extraordinary growth, it was an *effect* or unintended consequence of Congress's reform of Medicare in 1983.

It is not only natural but also intuitively appealing to assume that the paradigm shift from fee-for-service insurance to managed care was solely the result of the business community seeking to reduce costs by increasing managerial control and market mechanisms. "Firms face a very clear incentive structure: they must strive to maximize profits," as Paul Pierson and Jacob Hacker explain. "This conclusion does not rest on assumptions about individual greed, but on recognition that market systems are powerful mechanisms for inducing decision-makers to adopt profit-maximizing behavior."[6] Why, then, did the majority of businesses wait until the late 1980s and early 1990s to begin switching their employees into managed care (see table 7.5)? Why did they not begin the switch en masse in the late 1970s or early 1980s or even mid-1980s? Managed care had been an alternative since at least 1974, a year after President Nixon signed the HMO Act, which required businesses with more than twenty-five employees and that already offered health insurance to make HMOs available to their employees.[7]

Business's delayed switch to managed care suggests that existing market incentives were a necessary but not sufficient incentive for inducing such a paradigm shift in health insurance. The critical catalyst for making the market incentives sufficient had to come from another major actor—the single largest purchaser of hospital care: Medicare. As an institution, Medicare has been controlled by another institution: Congress. And according to J. K. Galbraith, "countervailing power has become in modern times perhaps the major domestic peacetime function of the federal government."[8]

Since Medicare and employers purchased their medical care from the same hospitals and doctors, one would expect that massive change to the former greatly affected (directly and indirectly) the cost-benefit calculations and policy decisions of the latter. It was the government, not business, that triggered the move from fee-for-service to managed care. The challenge is to explain precisely how and why. A parallel aim is to try to account for how individuals and institutions respond to changes in policy, recognizing that government reforms often reconfigure incentives other than those originally intended.

The government's reform of Medicare in 1983 led to the shift from fee-for-service insurance to managed care by doing two things. First, Medicare's new prospective payment system standardized hospital rates for the majority of hospital services and procedures. Referred to as diagnosis-related groups (DRGs), this standardization made hospital costs universally known. The PPS partly corrected the information asymmetry that had traditionally existed between hospitals and those who paid for their services: government and insurance companies. In time, many private payers employed Medicare's new payment system as an effective tool in controlling costs.[9]

Second, the PPS shifted financial power from hospitals to the government. When massive budget deficits emerged in the late 1980s, Congress could and did react by (among other measures) repeatedly reducing Medicare's reimbursement rates to the point where they became negative in 1990, 1991, and 1992 (explained later in the chapter). These reductions induced hospitals to vastly increase their cost-shifting to privately insured patients, thereby causing significant annual increases in health insurance premiums. Ultimately, businesses responded to the effects of government reform by rapidly moving the bulk of their employees out of fee-for-service plans and into various forms of managed care.

Why Medicare Needed Reform

By the advent of Ronald Reagan's new Republican administration in 1981, Medicare's rate of growth was clearly out of control and on an unsustainable trajectory (see figure 7.1, table 7.2). The structural concessions that policymakers made over Medicare in 1965, so that the program could finally overcome the AMA's political opposition, led to a very lucrative system for hospitals and doctors—so lucrative, in fact, that Medicare's costs quickly exploded. Policymakers had no choice but to reform Medicare in an effort to keep the program from going bankrupt.

As described in detail in chapter 6, financial flaws with Medicare arose soon after the program began operation. According to a report submitted to the Senate Finance Committee in spring 1966, the system for paying hospitals "contains no incentives whatsoever for good management and almost begs for poor management."[11] Robert Ball, commissioner of Social Security during Medicare's development and implementation, agreed: "After-the-fact reimbursement for hospital costs clearly was flawed, and within a couple of years I and other government officials were calling for some form of prospective payment."[12] Medicare's problem stemmed from its lack of cost-containment incentives; hospitals were neither penalized for cost increases nor rewarded for finding ways to control them.[13]

Figure 7.1
Medicare Enrollees and Payments, 1972-82

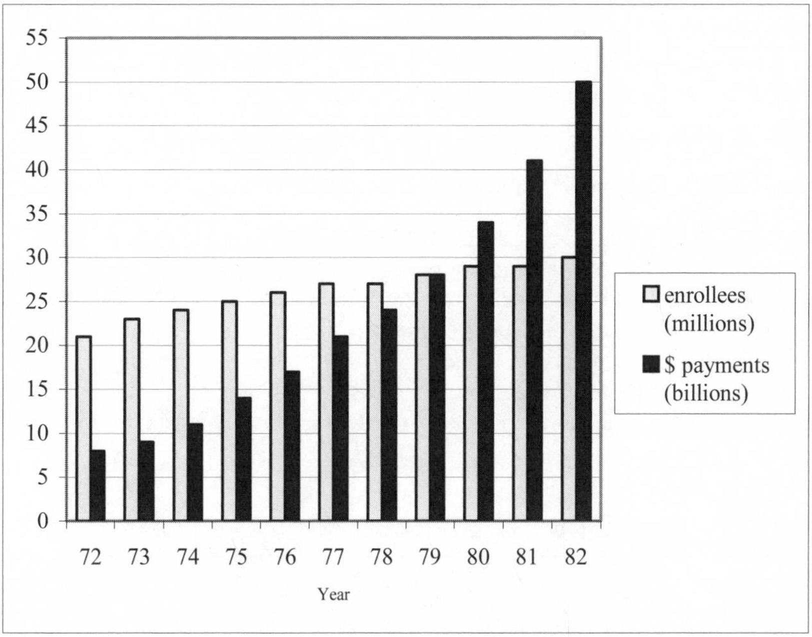

Source: Health Insurance Association of America, *Source Book of Health Insurance Data* (1992).

In rationalizing Medicare's hospital reimbursement scheme, the essential role of policy learning came by way of "applied federalism." In 1972, Congress had authorized the Department of Health and Human Services to conduct statewide experiments with different forms of hospital reimbursement.[14] By 1982, it was monitoring nine individual state experiments. One in New Jersey looked particularly promising with its novel use of diagnosis-related groups, designed in the late 1960s by Robert B. Fetter and John D. Thompson of Yale University. Their prospective system became the basis of Medicare's new PPS.[15] Louise Russell describes the plan's innovative approach: "The crucial features of Medicare's prospective payment system are that payment is prospective—rates are set before services are delivered—and that a single lump-sum rate pays for the entire hospital stay. . . . If the hospital can take care of the patient for less than the fixed rate, it keeps the profit. If not, it absorbs the loss."[16]

Changing Medicare payment from a retrospective to a prospective system was revolutionary.[17] Previously, doctors and hospitals often charged different payers different rates for the same procedure based on their ability to pay.

Government priorities so dominated the development of Medicare's PPS that there existed little interest group influence or congressional and media debate. Most members of Congress understood little to nothing of how the PPS worked.[19] But they voted for it because Medicare was approaching insolvency and because Democratic leaders in Congress piggybacked the plan onto vital Social Security legislation that had to pass for monthly OASDI checks to continue uninterrupted. Attaching Medicare reform to critical OASDI reform was a purely opportunistic, but effective, decision. A veto-proof bill emerged, immune from interest group influence due to its urgency.[19]

Public-Sector Reform as Catalyst for Private-Sector Reform

The PPS's phased-in approach had profound effects on hospitals. The PPS rationalized Medicare by categorizing all physician and hospital services, so that policymakers knew what medical care would cost *before* retirees received it. The new system established predetermined payment amounts for each patient through the use of diagnosis-related groups. If the hospital actually treated the patient for less than the DRG allotted, it kept the "savings" as profit. If, instead, the hospital incurred more costs than the DRG allotted, it had to absorb the loss.[20]

Table 7.1
Average Hospital Length of Stay for Adult Patients, 1980-88

Year	All Adults	Percentage Change	Medicare Adults	Percentage Change
1980	7.18	—	10.37	—
1981	7.21	0.4	10.36	-0.1
1982	7.16	-0.7	10.12	-2.3
1983	7.02	-2.0	9.68	-4.4
1984*	**6.66**	**-5.1**	**8.95**	**-7.5**
1985	6.55	-1.7	8.76	-2.1
1986	6.59	0.6	8.79	0.4
1987	6.64	0.8	8.88	1.0
1988	6.64	0.0	8.82	-0.7

Source: ProPAC, *Medicare and the American Health Care System, Report to the Congress* (Washington, D.C.: June 1991), 90.
* First full year of Medicare's PPS in operation (official starting date: October 1, 1983)

To cushion hospitals' transition from traditional retrospective reimbursement to a prospective system, first-year payments were based on each hospital's historical costs. This locked in what many already considered to be generous profit margins.[21] Hospitals responded by quickly reducing their average length of stay (table 7.1) and reaped huge windfall payments in excess of their already sizable pre-PPS profits:

Widely conceded "overpayment" in the first year of PPS created a situation in which margins were increasing as expenses per case were dropping, due to large reductions in length of stay. This not only made the first year a somewhat aberrant intervention, but also armed most hospitals with an unanticipated source of disposable funds, and probably altered expectations as well.[22]

Hospital administrators transformed their medical records departments—where accurate coding of patient records determined how much hospitals got paid or whether they got paid at all—with more personnel and improved technology. The cliché of choice became "PPS brought medical records out of the basement."[23] Massive change ensued. The Medicare hospital payment reforms "were the most drastic and far-reaching changes in Federal health policy since the passage of Medicare itself," notes David Smith, who has written the definitive account of the PPS's passage.[24]

In June 1984, Michael Bromberg, executive director of the Federation of American Hospitals, said as much in his testimony before Congress regarding Medicare's new PPS:

> The Medicare law that brought us prospective payment for the first time has clearly given us incentives 180 degrees different from any we have ever had, and we have responded. The change in behavior, not to have too many people employed per hospital simply because they are cost reimbursed, not to give extraordinary wage and benefit increases above the national average because [they are] cost reimbursed, to consider capital expenditures for the first time because they do increase operating costs and those are fixed for the first time, all the way down the line to trying to persuade the physicians to cooperate in lowering length of stay, doing more out-patient work, having arrangements with nursing homes and home health agencies and others for less expensive sites, and seeking discounts on supplies, all suddenly became real incentives for the first time.
>
> The most important point I can make today is that those incentives that I just outlined, every one of them, helps non-Medicare payers. In fact, those who predicted that we would simply take Medicare's price, absorb it, and raise our charges to everyone else were wrong.[25]

In May 1985, Bromberg reiterated his claim that Medicare's "Prospective Payment System is the most effective cost containment program ever enacted, successful beyond anyone's expectations."[26]

Everyone was initially pleased with Medicare's PPS. After its first year of operation, hospitals profited handsomely (figure 7.2), while overall Medicare and national health expenditures slowed (table 7.2). The new payment system appeared to be working to the financial good of both Medicare and the larger system of private health care.

Table 7.2
Total Medicare and National Health Expenditures (in billions), 1980-87

Year	National Health Expenditures	Percentage Change	All Medicare Expenditures	Percentage Change	Medicare Part A Payments	Percentage Change
1980	$249.1	—	$36.4	—	$25.4	—
1981	288.6	15.9	43.7	20.0	30.6	20.3
1982	323.8	12.2	51.2	17.3	35.7	16.5
1983	356.1	10.0	58.1	13.5	39.9	11.8
1984	387.0	8.7	64.8	11.5	44.5	11.7
1985	420.1	8.5	69.8	7.8	47.1	5.7
1986	452.3	7.7	75.8	8.5	49.2	4.6
1987	492.5	8.9	82.0	8.2	51.3	4.2
'80-83	—	12.7*	—	15.0*	—	16.2*
'84-87	—	8.5*	—	9.0*	—	6.5*

Source: ProPAC, *Medicare and the National Health Care System, Report to the Congress*
(Washington, D.C.: 1991), 12, 111.
* Annual average over the four-year period

Rising Budget Deficits and the Battle between Hospitals and Congress

The mutual admiration between Congress and the hospital industry over the success of the PPS deteriorated rapidly, however, when Congress turned to Medicare in 1986 as a means of addressing the nation's growing budget deficits.[27] The same Michael Bromberg, who just a year earlier had effusively praised Congress, now accused the Reagan administration and Congress of operating in "bad faith" and violating the PPS "contract":

> We are willing to accept our fair share of responsibility in any attempt to reduce the Federal Deficit. However, the cuts for the Medicare program proposed by the Administration once again go far beyond any sense of fairness and proportion. Consequently, health care providers will be asked to absorb much more than their fair share of the reductions.
>
> The Administration and Congress should note that the Medicare Hospital Insurance Trust Fund does not contribute to the Federal deficit. Payments to hospitals under Medicare do not come from general revenues; they are financed by a payroll tax. . . .
>
> If we had frozen payments to hospitals over the last 10 years what improvements would we have sacrificed? How many life-saving Intensive Care Units, or Cardiac Care Units or Neonatal Units would not exist today? What about technological advances like the CAT Scanner and MRI? Would we have the same quality and quantity of health care we enjoy today? Absolutely not!! . . .
>
> Hospitals understood the prospective payment law to be a contract. We have kept our part of the contract, and the system is working. However, if Congress unilaterally changes this contract by freezing or reducing hospital payments, then hospitals can hardly be expected to endorse the program.[28]

Although the PPS went a long way in correcting the information asymmetry between hospitals and Congress, conflict over information persisted and occasionally grew vitriolic. Hospitals started withholding requested financial information from Congress concerning their overall profit margins, concluding that Congress was only using it to justify further Medicare rate reductions. By 1988, Congress and the hospital industry were trading accusations of lying and fraud, as evidenced by the following exchange between Congressman Pete Stark (D-Calif.), chairman of the Subcommittee on Health of the Committee on Ways and Means, and Jack Owen, president of the American Hospital Association (AHA):

Chairman Stark: The railroads provide us better data than the hospitals. Think about that one for a minute.

Mr. Owen: I think the record will show that we have provided you with data in your committees whenever we could, on the basis of what is proprietary and what is not from the standpoint of the hospitals themselves.

Chairman Stark: There is no such thing as proprietary when you are asking for Federal dollars, my friend. That is when, as I say, if you do not like the system, you can drop out. . . .

Mr. Owen: I think the basic problem, though, is that it is not that no one wants to divulge it or let it go; it is just as you said earlier, you had some concern about the lack of trust, I guess. And I think there is a lack of trust in what has happened in this program well before you became chairman of the subcommittee. It started out in one fashion, and we hadn't even gone a year, and it was changed. There is a feeling by hospitals that all you really want data for—not you, personally, but all Congress wants data for—is so that they can take out more money to offset the budget deficits on the other side, and we are left with a patient who is lying in the hallway or who is bleeding and needs to be taken care of. That is a legitimate, I think, reason for being very cautious. If you want more data, then let's see something that indicates that we will be recognized for it, not rewarded for it, but recognized for it. It hasn't happened.

Chairman Stark: I suspect that is the concern, and if we were not providing the funds, that concern would bother me. But when we are constantly pressured by the same folks for more money—and you have seen the letters in my office, mostly from California hospitals, they just lie. They tell us they are going broke. And you and I both know that is just an unvarnished fabrication.

So you go in the same door you came out. The hospitals are concerned that we may use this data to cut funds. We are concerned that they may, in the most unconscionable way, use the data to create and fabricate situations which do not exist, in an effort to get more of the taxpayer's dollar.[29]

Congress ignored the hospital industry's complaints and repeatedly reduced Medicare's annual DRG-adjusted reimbursement increase (figure 7.2). As a result, more and more hospitals lost money on Medicare patients (table 7.3), particularly those with complicated diagnoses. And, in the process, hospitals began to experience greater pressure to increase revenue from other sources.

Hospitals' Increased Cost-Shifting to Privately Insured Patients

With consecutive annual decreases in inflation adjustments to their payments from Medicare, hospitals experienced greater pressure to increase revenue from other sources. By 1989, most hospitals were losing money on their Medicare patients (figure 7.2; table 7.3).[30] They responded largely by turning to privately insured patients to make up for their losses.[31]

Figure 7.2
Hospitals' Aggregate Profit Margin, 1984-92

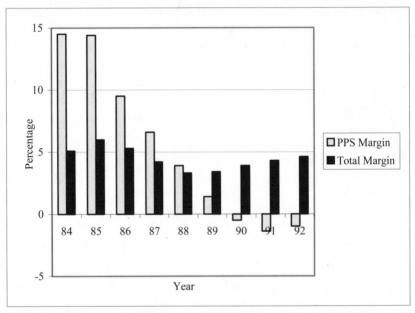

Source: ProPAC, *Medicare and the American Health Care System, Report to the Congress*
(Washington, D.C.: June 1995 and 1996), 55 and 68, respectively.

Table 7.3
Medicare's Aggregate PPS Margin (Profit or Loss)*
and Hospitals with Overall Medicare Losses by Percent, 1984-92

	1984	1985	1986	1987	1988	1989	1990	1991	1992
Margin*	14.5	14.0	9.5	6.6	3.9	1.4	-0.5	-1.4	-1.0
Percentage	16.8	18.8	32.3	39.8	46.1	51.8	56.7	60.8	60.0

Source: ProPAC, *Medicare and the American Health Care System, Report to the Congress*
(Washington, D.C.: June 1994 and 1996), 58 and 68, respectively.
* Medicare's PPS margin expressed as a percent increase = (revenues – costs) ÷ revenues

Table 7.4
Cost-Shifting: Hospital Losses and Gains as a Percentage of Costs, 1981-91

Year	Medicare Payments	Private Payments	Uncompensated ("Charity") Care
1981	-1.0%	5.0%	-3.3%
1983	-1.2	7.0	-3.6
1985	0.4	6.7	-4.4
1987	-0.7	8.2	-4.4
1989	-3.3	8.9	-4.4
1991	-4.4	11.6	-4.4

Source: ProPAC, *Report and Recommendations to the Congress* (Washington, DC: March 1994), 15.

Privately insured patients began to make up for the losses from Medicare and uncompensated care. Private payments as a percentage of total hospital gains more than doubled between 1981 and 1991 (table 7.4, figure 7.3). Businesses had long recognized the practice of cost-shifting prior to the PPS's implementation, but this form of cross-subsidization had traditionally remained at a modest enough level (approximately 5 percent) to avoid open conflict. Commercial insurers had also recognized the practice of cost-shifting prior to the PPS's implementation, as Donald M. Peterson, president of Benefit Trust Life Insurance and a representative of the Health Insurance Association of America, explained in congressional testimony:

> The existence of cost-shifting has become well-documented since our industry publicly identified the problem a couple of years ago. Cost-shifting totaled $5.8 billion in 1982. According to our latest estimates, the costs shift will grow to $8.4 billion in 1984. As a logical business practice, hospitals recoup reductions in Medicare and Medicaid reimbursement by inflating charges to private patients. Those who are insured face higher premiums.[32]

Evidence of extensive cost-shifting even came in the form of confession. In a written reply to a series of questions posed by the Senate Labor and Human Resources Committee, the American Hospital Association admitted that hospitals routinely shifted some of their costs to privately insured patients who then paid inflated bills:

> **Senate Committee**: How do hospitals finance uncompensated care?

> **AHA**: The vast bulk of uncompensated care is financed through charges paid by private insurers and individual patients. . . . A substantial part of the "cost shift" is the private sector's contribution to the cost of treating those individuals not covered—or inadequately covered—by public programs.[33]

There were consequences, however, for hospitals' creative accounting and the information asymmetry it prolonged.[34] The nation's top twelve corporate health insurance companies lost a combined $830 million in 1988, with only two carriers managing to post a profit.[35]

Figure 7.3
Private Insurance Gains and Public Losses as a Percentage of Hospital Costs, 1980-92*

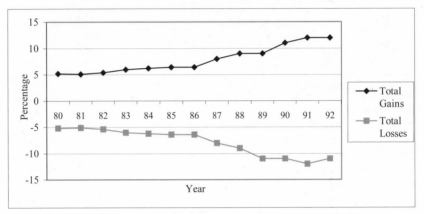

Source: ProPAC, *Medicare and the American Health Care System, Report to the Congress*
        (Washington, D.C.: 1994), 29.
* Gains and losses are the difference between the cost of providing care and the payment received.
Total gains (from private payers and operating subsidies above uncompensated care costs)
Total losses (from Medicare, Medicaid, other government payers, and uncompensated care)

With the rise of extensive cost-shifting, businesses concluded that their benefit-cost ratio for involvement in health insurance had fundamentally changed.[36] The problem of escalating private insurance premiums was not new, but cost-shifting greatly exacerbated it and led to unsustainable annual increases of between 20 and 40 percent between 1985 and 1990.[37] Hewitt Associates, a benefits consulting firm, identified cost-shifting as the single leading source of health plan premium increases in 1987 and 1988.[38] A survey of 1,500 corporate chief executives in 1990 showed that of the health care issues with which executives were *"very concerned,"* "rising health insurance premium costs" ranked first.[39] Ultimately, cost control in the public sector with Medicare reform fueled medical inflation in the private sector, which triggered the private sector's response: a massive switch to managed care (table 7.5).[40]

Table 7.5
Enrollment in Indemnity and Managed Care Health Insurance, 1989-95

Type of Coverage	1989	1993	1995
Indemnity (fee-for-service)	71%	49%	30%
Managed Care (HMO, PPO)	29%	51%	70%

Source: Employee Benefit Research Institute, *Sources of Health Insurance* (Washington, D.C.,
        February 1995).

Managed Care's Ascendance

The rationalizing politics that produced Medicare's prepaid formula for hospital reimbursement also contributed to the development of managed care.[41] "Policymakers hoped that similar analytic acumen and political ingenuity might devise a general cost containment strategy for health care that would forgo regulation in favor of the discipline of the medical marketplace," notes Lawrence Brown.[42]

Managed care's growth started slowly with President Nixon prodding Congress to pass the 1973 HMO Act. By July 1980, the government had qualified just 112 HMOs and only 4 percent of all U.S. citizens were members.[43] Policymakers learned that it was one thing to encourage an attractive business environment, but another to induce entrepreneurs to commit the enormous capital investments or "sunk costs" that managed care HMOs required to begin operation.[44] Eventually, due to cost-shifting from Medicare and the subsequent leap in health insurance premiums, enrollment in HMOs soared (figure 7.4).[45]

Figure 7.4
HMO Enrollment (in millions), 1970-92

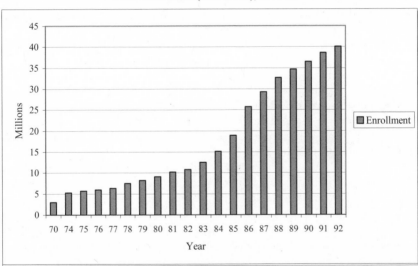

Source: Office of Health Maintenance Organizations, *National Census of Prepaid Health Plans* (Washington, D.C.: U.S. Department of HEW, 1978, 1979, and 1980; and Group Health Association of America, *Patterns of HMO Enrollment* (Washington, D.C.: 1992).

Managed care did nothing, however, to advance the goal of universal coverage. On the contrary, managed care and the Medicare reform that caused its rapid growth were primarily concerned with rationalizing health insurance for those who already had coverage. It would take another bout of medical inflation and a recession in the early 1990s to resurrect the issue of the uninsured.

Clinton's Effort: No Room to Maneuver

Harris Wofford's successful 1991 senatorial election in Pennsylvania[46] and Bill Clinton's presidential victory in 1992 provided a new window of opportunity for health care reform.[47] Universal coverage emerged as the defining characteristic of Clinton's proposal, the "organizing principle and the objective that shaped so much else in his health reform," argues Allen Schick. "Universal coverage meant that reform would be costly and controversial and would entail extensive regulation and redistribution."[48] Despite the elaborate policy innovations and complex arrangements in Clinton's proposal, the basic challenge was to extend coverage to the 15 percent of the population without stable coverage, while not alienating the insured 85 percent.

Because incrementally expanding current programs seemed impossible,[49] the only options for raising the necessary revenue were either increased taxes or employer mandates. Clinton chose the latter, to place most of the financing burden on employers due to the political impracticalities of raising taxes.[50] It was a logical choice, because the majority of employers provided health insurance.[51] And they largely subsidized those who did not, because medical providers simply shifted the costs of their uncompensated care to those with employer provided private insurance.[52] Besides, it was certainly not a new idea. President Nixon proposed an employer mandate twenty years earlier.[53]

The comprehensive plan that Clinton finally submitted to Congress on November 20, 1993 (introduced as S1757 and HR3600), constituted a gamble. The critical question was twofold: would the plan's rationalization and cost-containment aspects[54] generate sufficient revenue for financing universal coverage in a budget-neutral fashion, and would they survive politically? Congress would determine if the plan would remain intact. But the other half of the gamble—would Clinton's plan actually succeed as designed?—was addressed first by the Congressional Budget Office (CBO).

Since 1990, Congress's budgetary rules charged the CBO with estimating the projected cost of any new plan to make sure it did not add to the budget deficit.[55] The CBO finally reported on February 8, 1994, that Clinton's plan would actually *increase* the federal deficit by $74 billion in its first six years, instead of cutting it as the president had predicted.[56] The CBO concluded that Clinton's goals of universal coverage and cost-containment were very difficult, if not impossible, to reconcile. Moreover, the CBO could afford to consider the two goals independently, something Congress could not do.[57]

While the CBO argued that the budget could not afford Clinton's version of universal coverage, managed care's growth weakened the consensus that large-scale cost containment was imperative.[58] Reports in late 1993 that annual increases in health insurance premiums had dropped to their lowest level in twenty years (figure 7.5) undercut this key structural component of Clinton's argument—that his proposal's cost containment measures were fiscally necessary.[59] Analysts credited managed care for most of the decrease.[60]

Figure 7.5
Rate of Increase in Health Insurance Premiums, 1989-95

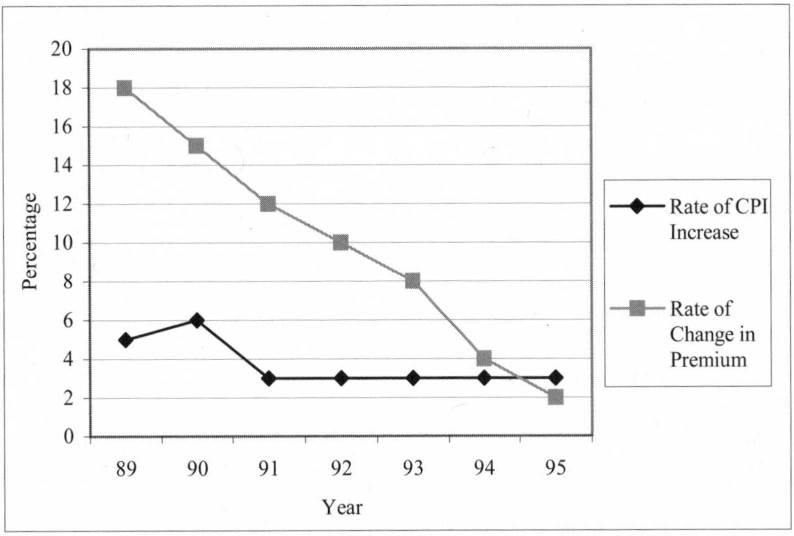

Source: Adapted and modified from Mercer/Foster Higgins; U.S. Bureau of Labor Statistics,
Nation's Business, July 1998, 20; Health Insurance Association of America/KPMG
Peat Marwick Survey, *Washington Post*, June 16, 1998, C3.

Exorbitant annual increases in health insurance premiums prior to 1993 contributed to the creation of a "policy window"[61] for reform. But as the inflation rate of premiums markedly decreased, so, too, did prospects for comprehensive reform.[62] Economic necessity may be the mother of policy innovation, but relative prosperity tends to foster a protection and maintenance of the status quo.

A Proliferation of Alternatives

The health care reform experience of 1993-94 underscored the crucial role of agenda setting.[63] Clinton could determine much of the agenda due to his role as president, but according to Schick, "The president's command of the agenda is accompanied by weakness in his ability to control legislative outcomes."[64] Once Clinton's proposal arrived in Congress as HR3600 and S1757, he could not rely on an institutionalized routine to constrain the free flow of participants and the number of plans they could propose. His proposal generated a proliferation of alternatives, all of which competed against each other in an environment that grew increasingly self-defeating with each new plan. The greater number of ever more complicated and poorly understood proposals drained political momentum and loyalty. These episodes stand in stark contrast to the experience of Medicare in 1965, and its epochal switch to a prospective system of payment (the PPS) in 1983. On both occasions, alternatives blended over time to the most

Chapter Seven

optimal scenario for policy change: one refined legislative proposal versus the status quo.

Table 7.6
Summary Comparison of Committee Health Care Reform Proposals, 1994

	Clinton's Health Security Act	House Education and Labor*	House Ways and Means^	Senate Labor†	Senate Finance°
Universal Coverage	- All Americans covered by 1998 through employer and individual mandates. - Subsidies for small businesses and low-income individuals.	- All Americans covered by 1998 through employer and individual mandates. - Subsidies for small businesses and low-income individuals.	- All Americans covered by 1998 through new Medicare Part C for uninsured. - Subsidies for small businesses and low-income individuals.	- All Americans covered by 1998 through employer and individual mandates. - Subsidies for small businesses and low-income individuals.	- No universal coverage or mandates. - Target of 95 percent insured by 2002. - Subsidies for low-income individuals.
Cost Control	- Spending caps on private insurance premiums. - Large Medicare cuts.	- Spending caps on private insurance premiums. -Large Medicare cuts. (Medicare not in committee jurisdiction.)	-Targets and limits on provider rates. - Large Medicare cuts begin 1996. - Private-sector limits begin 2001.	- Spending caps on private insurance premiums. Large Medicare cuts. (Medicare not in committee jurisdiction.)	No premium caps, rate limits, or "hard triggers" on private sector. Large Medicare cuts.
Financing	$103 billion in Medicare savings over five years from specific proposals. -Medicaid savings. -Tobacco tax. -Corporate tax.	- Financing not in committee jurisdiction.	- $110 billion in Medicare savings over five years, mostly from premium cap. -Medicaid savings. -Tobacco tax. -Corporate tax. -Revenue from non-enrolling employers.	- Financing not in committee jurisdiction.	$80-90 billion in Medicare savings over five years from specific proposals. -Tobacco tax. -Premium tax.

* Approved 26-17 (June 23, 1994) † Approved 11-6 (June 9, 1994).
^ Approved 20-18 (June 30, 1994) ° Approved 12-8 (July 2, 1994).

Unconstrained participation within Congress and the resulting proliferation of alternatives greatly enhanced the influence of both hostile interest group activity and what Jonathan Rauch refers to as "hyperpluralism."[65] Those interest groups opposed to employer mandates and additional corporate taxes no longer had to battle against a single, popular plan. Instead, they could easily exploit the confusion and lack of public understanding that grew as more alternatives arose in Congress. Also, the greater number of alternative plans made it unnecessary for interest groups to argue against the totality of any one plan. Rather, they could highlight specific components of numerous plans that, taken individually, proved to be immensely controversial and unpopular.

The lack of agenda-setting control and institutional restraint of participation became debilitating once Congress's formal process of deliberation began. Health care reform legislation was assigned to five standing committees: House Education and Labor, Energy and Commerce, and Ways and Means; and Senate Labor and Human Resources, and Finance (table 7.6).

Instead of trying to craft an alternative that was more likely to garner bipartisan consensus and support, "House and Senate leaders urged rank-and-file members to vote unpassable bills out of committee," notes Schick. "In health care reform, committee action was seen as an obstacle to legislation, not as a means of perfecting the measure and assembling votes needed for passage."[66] The House Energy and Commerce Committee failed to report out any bill. The two least bipartisan committees (House Education and Labor and Senate Labor and Human Resources) did produce alternative plans,[67] but they were politically unrealistic measures with notably even more generous (expensive) benefits and taxes than Clinton's original, politically unpassable design.[68] The Senate Finance Committee crafted a voluntary, phased-in plan that forsook universal coverage altogether, guaranteeing Clinton's veto should Congress pass it (an unlikely event).[69] Neither House nor Senate majority leaders used any of the three committees' bills as starting points in the drafting of their respective chambers' leading alternative proposals (submitted by Richard Gephardt on July 29 and George Mitchell on August 2, respectively).

Ways and Means' "Medicare Part C" Emerges as Leading Alternative

The Ways and Means Committee's final product became the House's leading alternative.[70] It bore explicit testimony to the influential role of lock-in effects associated with path dependency. Ways and Means was the only committee that crafted a new plan that both satisfied Clinton's requirement of universal coverage and received endorsement from House majority leaders. But rather than keeping numerous unpopular Clinton plan measures designed to facilitate universal coverage, such as "purchasing alliances," or building on the private sector's accumulated skills with managed care, Ways and Means stuck with the policymaking they knew best from thirty years of experience: Medicare. The bill's main component was "Medicare Part C" (table 7.7).

Table 7.7
Comparison of Administration, House, and Senate Reform Bills, 1994

	Clinton's Health Security Act	House Leadership Bill Gephardt/Foley*	Senate Leadership Bill Mitchell^
Universal Coverage	- All Americans covered by 1998 through employer and individual mandates. - Subsidies for small businesses and low-income individuals.	- All Americans covered by 1998 through employer and individual mandates. - Subsidies for low-income individuals. - Medicare Part C for those without private health insurance.	- If 95 percent of Americans not insured by 2000, then employer mandate for businesses with more than twenty-five workers would be "triggered" in 2002 in states with less than 95 percent coverage.
Cost Control	- Spending caps on private insurance premiums. - Large Medicare cuts.	- Spending caps on private insurance premiums, and Medicare Parts A, B, and new Part C enforced through limits on payment rates to physicians, hospitals, and other providers.	- No private-sector spending limits, but large Medicare cuts, and requirement that federal spending for health care not increase the deficit.
Financing	- $103 billion in Medicare savings over five years from specific proposals. - Medicaid savings. - Tobacco tax. - Corporate tax.	- $110 billion in Medicare savings over five years, mostly from premium cap. - Medicaid savings. - Tobacco tax. - Corporate tax. - Revenue from employers (w/100+ employees) who self-insure.	- $54 billion in Medicare savings over five years. - Medicaid savings. - Tobacco tax. - High-cost premium tax.

Source: The Henry J. Kaiser Family Foundation, "Health Reform Legislation: A Comparison of House and Senate Majority Leadership Bills," (August 1994).
* Introduced on July 29, 1994
^ Introduced on August 2, 1994

Medicare Part C, argues Max Heirich, was basically "a modified single-payer plan."[71] Ways and Means designed the program to cover the unemployed, part-time or seasonal workers, employees of small businesses (100 or fewer workers) that did not provide health insurance, and all others not eligible for employer-paid benefits.[72] Of the 124 million eligible individuals as of 1998, policymakers estimated that between 20 and 55 million would enroll in Medicare Part C, and that by 2004 the number could grow to as many as 100 million (with total Medicare beneficiaries, including retirees, constituting half of the entire population).[73] Medicare Part C explicitly fulfilled Robert Myers's prediction in 1970 that "the ultimate goal of the expansionists in medical care is relatively simple, but comprehensive: to provide Medicare benefits for the entire working population and retired populations and their dependents."[74]

Most policymakers, including Clinton, considered Medicare Part C absurd, anachronistic, and a political "non-starter," because its projected costs far exceeded the government's ability to raise the necessary revenue.[75] With the payroll tax exclusively devoted to existing programs, mainly Medicare and OASDI, policymakers were forced to pursue the only alternative means of financing— employer mandates—which was politically unacceptable.[76] Besides, the changes to the health care industry that Medicare Part C proposed aroused enough opposition from powerful interest groups—particularly the health insurance industry, doctors, and hospitals—that it had virtually no chance of passing.[77]

Final Stage: Legislative Paralysis

House and Senate leaders followed the committees' alternatives with two of their own (table 7.7). As previously mentioned, the Senate's version used little of the Finance and Labor and Human Resource Committee bills. It also did not achieve universal coverage except by way of phased-in "hard triggers" starting in 2002 if at least 95 percent of the population did not have insurance coverage. An unusual component of the Senate's plan would have mandated that individuals purchase health insurance, similar to many states' automobile insurance requirements.[78] As expected, corporate interest groups opposed Mitchell's new Senate bill, but so, too, did organized labor and other pro-reform groups.[79] When the mighty senior citizens' organization, the AARP, mildly endorsed the House and Senate leadership's new bills,[80] senior citizens undercut the AARP's influence by opposing its endorsement. The AARP received so many negative telephone calls following its endorsement that it was forced to discontinue its public advocacy of either bill.[81]

The House's alternative version of the Clinton plan, Ways and Means' Medicare Part C, inspired very little political confidence among rank-and-file members, because the scheme generated such intense interest group opposition and minimal public support. The plan required either a vast increase in taxation or employer mandates, both of which Congress lacked the sufficient number of supporters to pass.[82] According to Julie Rovner, "Although House Majority Leader Richard Gephardt was unsure he could find the votes to pass [Medicare Part C], Senate Majority Leader George Mitchell knew he could not even attempt such a proposal in the Senate."[83] According to Schick, "Gephardt's plan was no more passable than the Ways and Means bill on which it was based."[84]

Thus, House Democratic leaders—confirming off the record that they did not have the votes to pass any bill—deferred to the Senate and then postponed consideration of health care reform indefinitely.[85] The Senate followed suit on August 25 by recessing until September 12. Failing to resuscitate any consensus for reform in the interim, Mitchell sent a formal statement to Clinton on September 26, informing him that "health insurance reform cannot be enacted this year."[86]

Conclusion

In the 1980s, universal coverage was crowded out by policymakers' need for cost control through managed care and the rationalizing of Medicare's payment system (together with OASDI's contribution and benefit structure). In the 1990s, it was crowded out by two factors: (1) the accumulated costs of existing programs, *and* (2) the fragmented constellation of interest groups and organizations constituting the nation's patchwork health care system. Inherited financial obligations made reform for the purposes of universal coverage unacceptably expensive. With the payroll tax devoted to OASDI and Medicare, policymakers had to seek new policy paths for raising new revenues. They could not expand Medicare's coverage, nor could they establish new programs to cover the uninsured. Any alternative program unduly threatened established interests—employers, unions, the insurance industry, senior citizens, veterans, medical providers—that were loyal to their own public programs or private health insurance arrangements.

Thomas Jefferson once remarked, "Great innovations should not be forced on slender majorities."[87] Seconding Jefferson's claim, Paul Starr provides a lucid encapsulation of what has come to constitute *the* conventional wisdom for why health care reform failed in 1993-94:

> The collapse of health care reform in the first two years of the Clinton administration will go down as one of the great lost political opportunities in American history. It is a story of compromises that never happened, of deals that were never closed, of Republicans, moderate Democrats, and key interest groups that backpedaled from proposals they themselves had earlier cosponsored or endorsed. It is also a story of strategic miscalculation on the part of the president and those of us who advised him. . . . We made the error of trying to do too much at once, took too long, and ended up achieving nothing.[88]

Starr's argument is right, however, only in that it cannot be wrong. Yes, Clinton overreached and chose a fatal, one-time "all-or-nothing" strategy for a proposal already politically tenuous at best. But the conventional wisdom also begs a number of follow-up questions: Why didn't any compromises happen? Why weren't any deals closed? Why did Republicans, moderate Democrats, and key interest groups backpedal from earlier cosponsored or endorsed proposals?

Mark Rushefsky and Kant Patel point out that a variety of explanations for the defeat of health care reform in 1993-94 have been offered.[89] Some attribute the failure solely or partially to the institutional and structural features of the American political system. Others argue that attempts at health care reform failed because of business and various interest groups, the nature of class relations in American society, or President Clinton and his administration.[90]

While not denying the partial truth of these arguments, this chapter submits an alternative explanation for the failure of health care reform. It argues that the lock-in effects from path dependency provide a better explanation for why no compromises happened, why no deals were closed, and why Republicans, moderate Democrats, and key interest groups backpedaled from their earlier cosponsored or endorsed proposals.

To begin with, Clinton's plan was an ambitious effort to create a new path of policymaking. In an attempt to reorganize the nation's medical-industrial complex, the plan proposed an unworkable embrace of managed care with budget caps,[91] radical in its extension of government's regulatory power and difficult if not impossible to understand. The CBO deemed Clinton's plan to be a budgetary disaster.[92] So it reached Congress virtually at the outer fringes of political viability. "The Clinton administration and its friends tried to construct intergroup coalitions and grassroots campaigns on behalf of their vision of national health care reform," notes Theda Skocpol. "But there were organizational pitfalls, and even at their most effective, these efforts had pitifully scanty resources and faced great difficulties in mobilizing support for the President's reform plan as such."[93]

Incremental expansion had increased Medicare and particularly Social Security's generosity, but it limited the programs' range of potential protection and monopolized the tool it established for financing social insurance: the payroll tax. Consequently, policymakers of the 1990s were not able to add social insurance protections to an otherwise popular Social Security program as previous policymakers had. Instead, Clinton and others had to develop proposals that generated new and substantial revenues, harmonized inherited policy commitments (such as Medicare and Medicaid) with newly proposed ones, and reconciled various illogical arrangements produced by coexisting public and private health care systems (such as cost-shifting).

Blocked by the accumulated costs of Medicare and Social Security's OASDI program, Clinton was forced down a doomed path of policy innovation that included employer mandates,[94] health alliances, and explicit and implicit controls.[95] As Schick asserts, these few—yet salient—items are what principally derailed Clinton's proposed legislation.[96] David Brady and Kara Buckley argue that "considering both the preferences of legislators and the super-majority institutional arrangements in the Senate, the Clinton plan was doomed from the start."[97] Jacob Hacker concurs in this assessment:

> The Clinton proposal stood no chance of capturing the breadth of congressional support it needed. The proposal included a requirement that employers contribute to the costs of health insurance and a budget on national health spending—two measures that most conservative legislators opposed. As a result, it never had more than thirty Senate votes firmly on its side.[98]

Sallyanne Payton, who had been legal counsel to the Clinton White House for health care and a member of the Clinton Health Care Reform Task Force, maintains that the death knell for the Clinton proposal came when top officials of the largest corporations—whose health and benefit officers earlier had been supportive—did their own cost-benefit analysis of what they would gain and lose in terms of health benefits spending and taxes if the comprehensive insurance reform plan went into effect. They concluded it would cost them more than they would gain.[99] In effect, staying with the same private path made more sense than exiting to any different one.[100] "The Business Roundtable and the Chamber of Commerce withdrew their support for the legislative proposal in February, 1994," Heirich notes. "With this loss of support it became difficult to push even modified forms of the Clinton legislative proposal for health insurance reform through Congress."[101]

Following Clinton's failed effort to come up with a new policy-making path, the House Ways and Means Committee reverted to the only path it knew: Medicare. The committee's alternative plan, Medicare Part C, proposed to expand the coverage of Medicare, a program already considered to be in financial difficulty.[102]

Instead of Congress's plans evolving into more politically realistic improvements—based on leading innovations in both the public and private health care systems—they became successively weaker and more politically unrealistic. *Congressional Quarterly* described them as "patchwork measures" satisfying neither any conceivable majority in the House or the Senate nor either wing of the majority Democratic party.[103]

Congress's process of generating alternatives through its committee system became "anti-Darwinian," with each succeeding plan becoming less viable and likely to survive than what came before. Unable to expand existing programs or to forge new paths for reaching universal coverage, Congress produced increasingly unrealistic alternatives. The deliberative process ground to a halt without having produced any legislation that could pass.

In sum, policymakers could not find a politically satisfactory way of reconciling the enormous amount of existing financial obligations with new ones. The country's massive public debt made major new government commitments all but impossible.[104] Ambitious and unprecedented schemes, such as President Clinton's Health Security Act, proved futile in attempting to forge new policy paths around OASDI and Medicare. And old paths, such as the House leadership bill's "Medicare Part C," were hopelessly anachronistic. Policymakers could not expand existing programs, but neither could they successfully design, much less afford, any new ones.[105]

Notes

1. Paul Pierson, *Dismantling the Welfare State? Reagan, Thatcher, and the Politics of Retrenchment* (Cambridge: Cambridge University Press, 1994), 42-43.

2. As opposed to the prior method in which Medicare simply reimbursed hospitals and doctors at full cost for whatever services they provided to the program's beneficiaries. With its new PPS, Medicare switched to paying medical providers a preestablished amount of money for all services, procedures, and treatments.

3. "Health Care Cost Containment Strategies," *Hearing before the Committee on Labor and Human Resources*, United States Senate, 98th Congress, 2nd Session (June 21,

1984), 144; and "Payroll Taxes, Health Insurance, and SBA Budget Proposals," *Hearing before the Committee on Small Business*, House of Representatives, 101st Congress, 2nd Session (March 29, 1990), 4-9.

4. For example, see David F. Drake, "Managed Care: A Product of Market Dynamics," *The Journal of the American Medical Association* 277, no. 7 (February 19, 1997): 560-64.

5. Leiyu Shi and D. Singh, *Delivering Health Care in America: A Systems Approach* (Gaithersburg, Md.: Aspen Publishers, Inc., 1998), 299.

6. Jacob Hacker and Paul Pierson, "Business Power and Social Policy: Employers and the Formation of the American Welfare State" (paper presented at the Annual Meeting of the American Political Science Association, Washington, D.C., September 2000), 8.

7. See Lawrence D. Brown, *Politics and Health Care Organization* (Washington, D.C.: The Brookings Institution, 1983).

8. J. K. Galbraith, *American Capitalism: The Concept of Countervailing Power* (Boston: Houghton Mifflin, 1956), 136.

9. B. Goody et al., "New Directions for Medicare Payment Systems," *Health Care Financing Review* 16 (Winter 1994): 1-12.

10. Lawrence D. Brown, *New Policies, New Politics: Government's Response to Government's Growth* (Washington, D.C.: The Brookings Institution, 1983), 45: "Rationalizing politics are a government-led search for solutions to government's problems."

11. As quoted in Linda E. Demkovich, "Devising New Medicare Payment Plan May Prove Easier Than Selling It," *National Journal* 14, no. 47 (November 20, 1982): 1981.

12. Robert Ball, "Medicare's Roots: What Medicare's Architects Had in Mind," *Generations* 20 (Summer 1996): 7.

13. John Rapport, Robert Robertson, and Bruce Stuart, *Understanding Health Economics* (Rockville, Md.: Aspen Systems Corporation, 1982), 330.

14. Carolyne K. Davis, "The Federal Role in Changing Health Care Financing, Part II," *Nursing Economics* (September/October 1983): 98-104.

15. "Fetter, Thompson: Inventors of DRG's Look at PPS Now," *Hospitals* (July 5, 1992): 137.

16. Louise B. Russell, *Medicare's New Hospital Payment System: Is It Working?* (Washington, D.C.: The Brookings Institution, 1989) 7-9: "The foundation for Medicare's prospective rates is a patient classification system called Diagnosis-Related Groups (DRGs), which sorts patients into groups according to medical condition. . . . Groups were included in the new set only if they made medical sense to an advisory panel of physicians and differed significantly in cost from other groups. The prospective rate is the same for every patient in a given group, regardless of how long the patient stays in the hospital or what else is done during the stay."

17. See Rosemary Stevens, *In Sickness and in Wealth: American Hospitals in the Twentieth Century* (New York: Basic Books, 1989) 322-27.

18. John Iglehart, "Health Policy Report," *New England Journal of Medicine* 23 (June 9, 1983): 1429: "A remarkable reality of the process in both chambers was how few legislators were actually involved in designing the legislation. For the most part, professional staff members made the key decisions."

19. Timothy Clark, "Congress Avoiding Political Abyss By Approving Social Security Changes," *National Journal* 15 (March 19, 1983): 611-15. See also, Paul Light, *Artful Work: The Politics of Social Security Reform* (New York: Random House, 1985), 3: "This is a story about a legislative miracle. Under extreme time pressure in 1983 (and

largely because of it), Congress and the President finally passed a Social Security rescue bill. Two years in the making, the legislation arrived just moments before the Social Security trust fund was to run dry. Without the $170-billion package of tax increases and benefit cuts, millions of checks would have been delayed."

20. "Medicare's Prospective Payment System: Strategies for Evaluating Cost, Quality, and Medical Technology," Office of Technology Assessment, United States Congress (Washington, D.C.: GPO, 1985): 3.

21. "Medicare's Prospective Payment System," 3.

22. Robert F. Coulam and Gary L. Gaumer, "Medicare's Prospective Payment System: A Critical Appraisal," *Health Care Financing Review, 1991 Annual Supplement*, U.S. Department of Health and Human Services, Health Care Financing Administration (Baltimore, 1991): 46.

23. David Burda, "What We Have Learned from DRG's," *Modern Healthcare* (October 4, 1993): 44.

24. David Smith, *Paying for Medicare: The Politics of Reform* (New York: Aldine de Gruyter, 1992).

25. "Health Care Cost Containment Strategies," *Hearing Before the Committee on Labor and Human Resources*, United States Senate, 98th Congress, 2nd Session (June 21, 1984): 192.

26. "Issues Relating to Medicare Hospital Payments," *Hearing Before the Subcommittee on Health of the Committee on Ways and Means*, House of Representatives, 99th Congress, 1st Session (May 14, 1985): 158.

27. See Dennis Ippolito, *Uncertain Legacies: Federal Budget Policy from Roosevelt through Reagan* (Charlottesville: University Press of Virginia, 1990), chs. 6 and 7; and Joseph White and Aaron Wildavsky, *The Deficit and the Public Interest* (Berkeley: University of California Press, 1989), chs. 19 and 21.

28. "1987 Medicare Budget Issues," *Hearing before the Subcommittee on Health of the Committee on Ways and Means*, House of Representatives, 99th Congress, 2nd Session (March 6, 1986): 338-39.

29. "Status of the Medicare Hospital Prospective Payment System," *Hearing Before the Subcommittee on Health of the Committee on Ways and Means*, 100th Congress, 2nd Session (March 1, 1988): 83-84.

30. See S. Guterman, S. Altman, and D. Young, "Hospitals' Financial Performance in the First Five Years of PPS," *Health Affairs* 9 (1990): 125-34; and S. Altman and J. Ashby, "The Trend in Hospital Output and Labor Productivity, 1980-89," *Inquiry* 29 (Spring 1992): 80-92.

31. See Jack Needleman, "Cost-Shifting or Cost-Cutting: Hospital Responses to High Uncompensated Care" (Cambridge, Mass.: Malcolm Wiener Center for Social Policy, John F. Kennedy School of Government, Harvard University, 1994); and Michael Morrisey, Cost Shifting in Health Care (Washington, D.C.: AEI Press, 1994).

32. "Health Care Cost Containment Strategies," *Hearing before the Committee on Labor and Human Resources*, 148. See also, Demkovich, "Devising New Medicare Plan May Prove Much Easier Than Selling It," 1984.

33. "Health Care Cost Containment Strategies," *Hearing Before the Committee on Labor and Human Resources*, 187.

34. Dean C. Coddington, David J. Keen, and Keith D. Moore, "Cost Shifting Overshadows Employers' Cost-Containment Efforts," *Business & Health* (January 1991): 45-51.

35. See R. Donahue, "Top 12 Health Insurers Lose $830 Million in 1988," *National Underwriter Life & Health/Financial Services* (1989): 1,4; and R.C. Coile, "The Megatrends-and the Backlash," *Health Care Forum Journal* (March/April 1990): 38.

36. David Burda and Cathy Tokarski, "Hospitals Are under Pressure to Justify Cost Shifting: But Some Payers Are Rejecting Hospitals' Excuses and Are Demanding Data," *Modern Healthcare* (November 12, 1990): 28-36

37. See "Payroll Taxes, Health Insurance, and SBA Budget Proposals," *Hearing before the Committee on Small Business*, House of Representatives, 101st Congress, 2nd Session (March 29, 1990): 4-9.

38. See Dean Coddington, David Keen, and Keith Moore. *The Crisis in Health Care* (San Francisco, Calif.: Jossey-Bass Publishers, 1990), 103; and G. Ruffenach, "Health Insurance Premiums to Soar in '89," *Wall Street Journal*, October 23, 1989, B12.

39. "1990 National Executive Poll on Health Care Costs/Benefits," *Business & Health* (April 1990): 26.

40. See Cathie J. Martin, "Nature or Nurture? Sources of Firm Preference for National Health Reform," *American Political Science Review* 89, no. 4 (December 1995): 898-914. For further evidence and explanation for businesses responding to cost-shifting by switching to managed care, see Coddington, Keen, and Moore, "Cost Shifting Overshadows Employers' Cost-Containment Efforts"; and Coddington, Keen, and Moore, *The Crisis in Health Care.*

41. Tom James III and David B. Nash, "Health Maintenance Organizations: A New Development or the Emperor's Old Clothes?" in *Readings in American Health Care*, ed. William G. Rothstein (Madison: University of Wisconsin Press, 1995), 268: Managed care is "an organized system which accepts responsibility and risk for both the financing and delivery of comprehensive health care services to a defined voluntarily enrolled population for a fixed monthly prepaid amount." It primarily represented a strategic response by employers to increased cost-shifting.

42. Brown, *Politics and Health Care Organization*, vii, 15. The term "health maintenance organization" was coined by Paul Ellwood, a health policy scholar, in 1970 in his article: "Health Maintenance Strategy," *Medical Care* 291 (1971): 250-56. Managed care, or prepaid group practice, originated in 1929 with the Elk City Cooperative in Elk City, Oklahoma, and the Ross-Loos Clinic in Los Angeles. For an account of early managed care programs prior to 1973, see W. MacColl, *Group Practice and Prepayment of Medical Care* (Washington, D.C.: Public Affairs Press, 1966), ch. 2. For more on administrative aspects of HMOs, see P. Moore, *Evaluating Health Maintenance Organizations* (New York: Quorum Books, 1991).

43. "HMO's," Health Care Financing Administration, 2. See also, "Factors that Impede Progress in Implementing the Health Maintenance Organization Act of 1973" (Washington, D.C.: GAO, September 3, 1976).

44. Brown, *Politics and Health Care Organization*, 444: "Under the spell of the analysts' code words, policymakers failed to anticipate how difficult it might prove to be to build HMO's by means of public policy. As the difficulties became clear in the course of trial and errors, critics—including some of the policy analysts who had originally sold the proposal in Washington—concluded that politicians had taken up an excellent idea and somehow managed to ravish it."

45. Moore, *Evaluating Health Maintenance Organizations*, 16. The number of HMOs more than doubled in just four years from 306 in 1984 to 653 by 1988.

46. For more on how Wofford's victory significantly raised the political profile of health care reform, see Haynes Johnson and David Broder, *The System: The American Way of Politics at the Breaking Point* (Boston: Little Brown, 1996), 58-62; and Thomas

Mann and Norman Ornstein, *Intensive Care: How Congress Shapes Health Policy* (Washington, D.C.: The Brookings Institution, 1995), 182-83.

47. Henry J. Aaron, ed., *The Problem That Won't Go Away: Reforming U.S. Health Care Financing* (Washington, D.C.: The Brookings Institution, 1996); Jacob S. Hacker, *The Road to Nowhere: The Genesis of President Clinton's Plan for Health Security* (Princeton, N.J.: Princeton University Press, 1997); Johnson and Broder, *The System*; Nicholas Laham, *A Lost Cause: Bill Clinton's Campaign for National Health Insurance* (Westport, Conn.: Praeger, 1996); and Theda Skocpol, *Boomerang: Health Care Reform and the Turn Against Government* (New York: W. W. Norton & Company, 1996).

In *Health Affairs* 14 (Spring 1995), see: Hugh Heclo, "The Clinton Health Plan: Historical Perspective," 86-98; James Mongan, "Anatomy and Physiology of Health Reform's Failure," 99-101.

In *Journal of Health Care Politics, Policy & Law* 20 (Summer 1995), see: Frank R. Baumgartner and Jeffery C. Talbert, "From Setting a National Agenda on Health Care to Making Decisions in Congress," 437-45; David Brady and Kara Buckley, "Health Care Reform in the 103d Congress," 447-54; Cathie J. Martin, "Stuck in Neutral: Big Business and the Politics of National Health Reform," 431-36; James A. Morone, "Nativism, Hollow Corporations, and Managed Competition," 391-98; V. Navarro, "Why Congress Did Not Enact Health Care Reform," 455-62; Bert Rockman, "The Clinton Presidency and Health Care Reform," 399-402; Steven Smith, "Commentary—The role of Institutions and Ideas in Health Care Policy," 385-89; Sven Steinmo and Jon Watts, "It's the Institutions, Stupid! Why Comprehensive National Health Insurance Always Fails in America," 329-72; Joseph White, "Commentary-The Horses and the Jumps: Comments on the Health Care Reform Steeplechase," 373-83.

See also, Martha Derthick, "Endless Ramifications," *Washington Post*, August 31, 1994, A25; John Judis, "Abandoned Surgery: Business and the Failure of Health Care Reform," *American Prospect* 21 (Spring 1995): 65-73; A. Schick, "How a Bill Did Not Become a Law," in *Intensive* Care, ed. Mann and Ornstein, 227-72; and P. Starr, "What Happened to Health Care Reform?" *American Prospect* 20 (Summer 1995): 20-31.

48. Schick, "How a Bill Did Not Become a Law," 231.

49. For more on the extreme difficulty of expanding existing programs, see Richard Himelfarb's definitive work on the 1988-89 Medicare Catastrophic Coverage Act debacle, *Catastrophic Politics* (University Park, Penn.: Pennsylvania State University Press, 1995). In this instance, Congress attempted to increase Medicare's coverage to include previously uncovered "catastrophic" expenses through progressive financing solely from retirees, instead of regressive taxation primarily on the working population. Lock-in effects associated with Medicare made exiting to this type of new path politically unpalatable. According to Himelfarb: "The key to understanding the MCCA's passage and eventual repeal lies in the decision of Congress to depart from previous practice in the area of social insurance policy-making. Specifically, in an attempt to expand Medicare in a deficit-neutral manner without imposing costs on younger generations, the new program imposed all costs on elderly beneficiaries themselves. In addition, costs were distributed in a progressive manner, in order to avoid burdening low-income senior citizens and to establish a precedent for future policy-making in social-insurance programs."

50. See Marie Gottschalk, *The Shadow Welfare State: Labor, Business, and the Politics of Health Care in the United States* (Ithaca, N.Y.: Cornell University Press, 2000), 152-54.

51. Gottschalk, *The Shadow Welfare State*, 65-66, 159.

52. J. Kosterlitz, "Kennedy's New Task," *National Journal* 19 (March 14, 1987): 608.

53. Gottschalk, *The Shadow Welfare State*, 65, n. 1.

54. The controversial aspects included employer mandates, massive purchasing cooperatives, caps on insurance premiums, reductions in future Medicare spending, increased tobacco taxes, community rating of individuals' insurance premiums instead of experience rating, and corporate taxes for those companies that self-insured.

55. Joseph White, "Budgeting and Health Policymaking," in *Intensive Care*, ed. Mann and Ornstein, ch. 3.

56. Congressional Budget Office, *Analysis of the Administration's Health Proposal* (Washington, D.C., 1994): 35; "CBO Turns Budget Spotlight on Health-Care Overhaul," *CQ Weekly Report* 52 (February 12, 1994): 290-91; "Health Plan Will Swell Deficit, Hill Office Says," *Washington Post*, February 9, 1994, A1: "Robert D. Reischauer, director of the nonpartisan [CBO], said the chief reason is that health insurance premiums would cost 15 percent more than the administration has estimated. As a result, the government would be required to pay higher subsidies to help low-income people and small businesses buy insurance."

57. No plan with universal coverage as one of its main goals could be financially viable without additional revenues gained from cost control. And no interest existed for cost control as an end in itself.

58. "Medical Costs Are Increasing at a Low Rate: Studies Show Slowest Pace in 20 Years," *Wall Street Journal*, July 14, 1994, 2. See also, Paul Starr, "What Happened to Health Care Reform?" *American Prospect* 20 (Winter 1995): 22: "With unemployment down, Americans were worrying less about their jobs and health coverage and more about crime. As health care inflation eased [by late 1993] primarily because inflation was generally under control, businesses worried less about health care cost containment and more about the political implications of an expansion of government authority. . . . Overconfident about the momentum of reform, we misjudged the health care politics of 1993 as a change in the climate when it was only a change in the weather."

59. "Health Care Cost Growth Slowing Down: Trend May Dampen Prospects for Reform," *Washington Post*, December 22, 1993, A1. See also, "Rethinking the Goals of Clinton Reform Plan: Survey Indicates Big Strides in Group Health Cost Control," *Business Insurance* (October 25, 1993): 2.

60. "Health Care Cost Growth Slowing Down," and "Rethinking the Goals of Clinton Reform Plan."

61. John Kingdon, *Agendas, Alternatives, and Public Policies* (Boston: Little, Brown & Company, 1984).

62. See Jacob Hacker, "National Health Care Reform: An Idea Whose Time Came and Went," *Journal of Health Politics, Policy and Law* 21 (Winter 1996): 647-96.

63. See Frank R. Baumgartner and Bryan D. Jones, *Agendas and Instability in American Politics* (Chicago: University of Chicago Press, 1993); and Gary Mucciaroni, *Reversals of Fortune: Public Policy and Private Interests* (Washington, D.C.: The Brookings Institution, 1995).

64. Schick, "How a Bill Did Not Become a Law," 230.

65. Jonathan Rauch, *Demosclerosis: The Silent Killer of American Government* (New York: Times Books, 1994). For more on Rauch's argument explicitly applied to the health care reform debate, see Schick, "How a Bill Did Not Become a Law," 238-39: "Health care reform fell victim to hyperpluralism in American politics. This condition refers to the vast growth in the number of interest groups, . . . trade associations and 'Washington representatives" seeking to influence national policy. Growth has occurred through a fissionlike process in which specialized interests separate from broader groups.

In some circumstances the fracturing of interests can facilitate compromise and mobilization of support for controversial measures. . . . In health care reform, however, the comprehensive sweep of the legislation complicated the politics of providing exclusive benefits to a relatively narrow band of groups. The legislation significantly affected just about every interest group with a stake in health care. This was not a narrow-gauge measure that benefited some while not affecting many others. It forced just about everyone to choose sides. The final lineup was heavily weighted against the Clinton plan as well as against others devised by Democratic leaders in Congress."

66. Schick, "How a Bill Did Not Become a Law," 258: "These legislative chores would be performed, the leaders promised, after the committees were done and not before."

67. "Summary: Senate Committee on Labor and Human Resources Health Care Reform Mark" (June 9, 1994), from the Office of Senator Edward M. Kennedy.

68. "Key Committees Bear Down on Overhaul Proposals," *CQ Weekly Report* (June 11, 1994): 1521-22: "If the larger effort fails, the [Senate Labor] committee and the Massachusetts Democrat [Edward Kennedy] will share the blame for failing to craft a bill that could win GOP support."

69. "White House Attacks Critics on Health Care," *Wall Street Journal*, July 25, 1994, 2: "The Clinton administration [is] portraying more incremental, competing plans as ineffective and less than true reform. . . . [Vice President] Mr. Al Gore said, 'Plans that do not provide universal coverage do not work.'"

70. See "Summary: House Democratic Healthcare Reform Bill as of August 10, 1994," *Federal Health Update* (August 10, 1994).

71. Max Heirich, *Rethinking Health Care* (Boulder, Colo.: Westview Press, 1998), 120.

72. Committee on Ways and Means, *Health Care Reform: Chairman's Mark* (June 10, 1994), 149-59.

73. Committee on Ways and Means, *Health Care Reform*, 149-59.

74. Robert Myers, *Expansionism in Social Insurance* (London: Institute of Economic Affairs, 1970), 22. Robert Myers was the Social Security Administration's chief actuary from 1938 to 1970.

75. Johnson and Broder, *The System*, 621: "The bill [Medicare Part C], which envisaged a much larger role for the federal government than anything the President had in mind, became the main vehicle in the House—and could not be passed." See also, "Plan to Expand Medicare Sparks Health Skirmish," *Los Angeles Times*, July 23, 1994, A1; "Medicare C: A Massive New Program," *Washington Post*, July 1, 1994, A14; "Medicare as Safety Net?" *American Medical News* (August 15, 1994): 3; and "Plan to Expand Medicare Pains the Health Industry," *Washington* Post, August 5, 1994, A19.

76. See "Democratic Governors Want Reform, but not Employer Mandate," *American Medical News* 37 (August 1, 1994): 6; "Democrats Band Together to Repel Assault on Employer Mandate," *CQ Weekly Report* 52 (June 18, 1994): 1615-619.

77. "Democratic Governors Want Reform, but not Employer Mandate, nn. 48 and 49. See also, "Health Care Debate Promises 'Fire and Light,'" *National Underwriter* 98 (August 8, 1994): 9.

78. Congressional Budget Office, *A Preliminary Analysis of Senator Mitchell's Health Proposal* (Washington, D.C.: GPO, August 9, 1994), 6: "A mandate requiring that individuals purchase health insurance would be an unprecedented form of federal action. The government has never required individuals to purchase any good or service as a condition of lawful residence in the United States. Therefore, neither existing budgetary

precedents nor concepts provide conclusive guidance about the appropriate budgetary treatment of a mandate."

79. "Labor Turns Up Heat on Senate Health-Care Bill," *Wall Street Journal*, August 5, 1994, 3; "Clinton Move on Health Divides Hill Coalitions," *Washington Post*, August 5, 1994, A1.

80. AARP Press Release, "It's Time for Health Care Reform" (August 11, 1994).

81. AARP Interoffice Memorandum (August 12, 1994): "This is an update on a sample of about 250 Friday phone calls. As we all know, the vast majority of calls are negative. . . . Many of those who call are extremely angry and upset. Some start crying; others resort to profanities that would 'make a sailor blush.'" See also, "Rogue Lobbyists," *Investor's Business Daily* (August 1, 1994): A2: "The AARP's professional staff vigorously advocates a new health entitlement. But membership isn't so sure. One poll found more than three out of four members opposed the Clinton plan."

82. "Part C: Defending the Controversial," *Health Line* (August 5, 1994); "House Delays Health Care Debate as Leaders Plot Strategy," *CQ Weekly Report* 52 (August 13, 1994): 2349-53; and "Mitchell Trying to Find a Graceful Exit," *CQ Weekly Report* 52, (September 24, 1994): 2693-95.

83. Julie Rovner, "Congress and Health Care Reform 1993-94," in *Intensive Care*, ed. Mann and Ornstein, 218.

84. Schick, "How a Bill Did Not Become a Law," 264.

85. Schick, "How a Bill Did Not Become a Law," 220; "House Letting Senate Go First: Many Democrats Happy," *New York Times*, August 5, 1994, A1; and "Doubt Surfaces on Bill Passage as Senate Struggle Continues," *CQ Weekly Report* 52 (August 20, 1994): 2458.

86. "For Health Care, Time Was a Killer," *New York Times*, August 29, 1994, A1; "Health Care Reform: The Collapse of a Quest," *Washington Post*, October 11, 1994, A6.

87. As quoted by John F. Kennedy in Arthur M. Schlesinger Jr., *A Thousand Days: John F. Kennedy in the White House* (Boston: Houghton Mifflin, 1965), 709.

88. Starr, "What Happened to Health Care Reform?" 20, 31.

89. Mark E. Rushefsky and Kant Patel, Politics, *Power & Policymaking: The Case of Health Care Reform in the 1990s* (New York: M. E. Sharpe, 1998), 68-69.

90. Rushefsky and Patel, *Power & Policymaking*, 68-69. For comprehensive author citations, see n47 of this chapter. For institutional explanations for the defeat of health care reform in 1993-94, see Steinmo and Watts 1995; White 1995; Smith 1995; Morone 1995. For interest group explanations, see Martin 1995; Baumgartner and Talbert 1995; Judis 1995. For class explanations, see Navarro 1995. Finally, for explanations that stress President Clinton and his administration's strategic shortcomings, see Rockman 1995.

91. See Theodore Marmor, *The Politics of Medicare*, 2d ed. (New York: Aldine de Gruyter, 2000), 167.

92. See Skocpol, *Boomerang*, 67-68; and Hacker, *The Road to Nowhere*, 124.

93. Skocpol, *Boomerang*, 90.

94. See Lewin-VHI, "Expanding Insurance Coverage without a Mandate," prepared for the Health Care Leadership Council (Lewin-VHI, Inc., May 19, 1994).

95. See Richard Scott et. al, *Institutional Change and Healthcare Organizations: From Professional Dominance to Managed Care* (Chicago: University of Chicago Press, 2000), 232.

96. Schick, "How a Bill Did Not Become a Law," 230.

97. See Brady and Buckley, "Health Care Reform in the 103rd Congress: A Predictable Failure," 447-54.

98. Hacker, *The Road to Nowhere*, 174.

99. See Sallyanne Payton, "The Politics of Comprehensive National Health Reform: Watching the 103rd and 104th Congress," in *Health Policy*, ed. Max Heirich and Marilynn M. Rosenthal (Boulder, Colo.: Westview Press, 1998).

100. See Gottschalk, *The Shadow Welfare State*, 153.

101. Heirich, *Rethinking Health Care*, 121.

102. Even ardent supporters of achieving universal coverage through Medicare acknowledged its political impracticality. See Morone, "Nativism, Hollow Corporations, and Managed Competition," 397: "There is only one large-scale, politically plausible, American [hope for] health care reform: Medicare. Expanding Medicare has a constituency. The program is already very popular. It is simple to understand. The infrastructure is in place. . . . However, expanding Medicare is a fast-fading possibility."

103. "Gibbons' Patched-Together Health Bill Now Faces Test on the Floor," *CQ Weekly Report* 52 (July 2, 1994): 1793.

104. Hacker, *The Road to Nowhere*, 181.

105. For more on this dilemma, see Jacob Hacker and Theda Skocpol, "The New Politics of U.S. Health Policy," *Journal of Health Politics, Policy and Law* 22 (April 1997): 315-38.

CHAPTER EIGHT

Conclusion

The full importance of an epoch-making idea is often not perceived in the generation in which it is made: it starts the thoughts of the world on a new track, but the change of direction is not obvious until the turning-point has been left some way behind. . . . For a new discovery is seldom fully effective for practical purposes till many minor improvements and subsidiary discoveries have gathered themselves around it.

—**Economist Alfred Marshall**
Principles of Economics (1890)

The United States remains the only Western nation without universal health insurance coverage. As the preceding analysis illustrates, there are two major factors that help to explain this distinct anomaly. First, the success policymakers had in passing a generous Medicare program, along with incrementally expanding the nation's core social insurance program—old age, survivors and disability insurance (OASDI)—eventually led to a cost explosion that prevented Social Security from fulfilling universal coverage.[1] As a result, social insurance reached its zenith in the mid-1970s, a decade after Medicare's enactment and shortly after both OASDI benefits were increased by an unprecedented 20 percent and Medicare coverage was extended to recipients of disability insurance. Since that time, policymakers have been almost exclusively preoccupied with finding ways to control the two programs' persistent financial escalation.[2] This obstacle to universal coverage is a relatively familiar one to most observers and generates minimal disagreement.

The second factor is something of a corollary to the first, but much more open to challenge—particularly by those who are impassioned advocates of social insurance. Over time, both the private sector's path of tax-subsidized, employer-provided health insurance *and* the public path of different government health insurance programs for targeted "clients" or segments of the population crowded out alternative paths to universal coverage (eventually cutting them off entirely).[3]

139

Once the payroll tax became solely devoted to covering Social Security and Medicare's rapidly increasing costs, policymakers grew convinced that they could not raise it for any additional commitments. They chose, instead, to pursue alternative financing proposals for increasing health insurance coverage. All of them proved politically futile because any substantial broadening of the government's role in health insurance after the mid-1970s either threatened entrenched, private interests (such as the insurance industry) or risked encouraging employers to discontinue providing coverage for their employees.

The Equilibrium: Various Constituencies with Separate Loyalties

Just as policymakers' expansion of OASDI secured a public path for retirement support, over time collective bargaining secured a private path for health insurance. By reducing uncertainty and promoting routine patterns of retirement and medical care provision, the two paths became locked in (albeit with private health insurance falling short of universal coverage). Individuals and organizations continually found it more profitable in the short run to adjust their behavior to the existing paths than to try pursuing an alternative one. Economists refer to this dynamic as the "quasi-irreversibility of investments," wherein established programs "generate powerful inducements that reinforce their own stability and further development."[4]

An equilibrium developed in society with individuals incorporating OASDI into their retirement plans, while relying on private health insurance for their medical care until they retired.[5] The equilibrium was self-reinforcing because it offered individuals and organizations big advantages for choosing to join it and punitive costs for deviating from it. So the equilibrium was continually reinforced and augmented, not because it was imposed, but because it arose from large groups in society.[6]

The popularity of Social Security's OASDI program made it possible in 1965 for policymakers to address various gaps in private health insurance. With Medicare, they were able to overcome the AMA's hitherto successful opposition to public health insurance by incrementally expanding Social Security. As a programmatic institution, OASDI opened a number of policy opportunities for public health insurance that previously did not exist. Organizations such as the Social Security Administration and organized labor took advantage of these opportunities, using incremental expansion as a strategy to pass Medicare.[7]

But Medicare's passage solidified the incremental approach of having separate public programs and private health insurance arrangements for individual constituencies; each of which responded by generating distinct loyalties to their own programs or arrangements. Every new program added another formidable constituency opposed to exiting to any new, comprehensive scheme for universal coverage, because the adaptation costs involved in exiting rose exponentially (as did the constituencies' fears that radical change might result in benefits being sacrificed for the utilitarian good of covering everyone).

Incremental expansion also had a negative result that surfaced only after OASDI and Medicare stalled in the early 1970s. Once the programs' returns ceased to increase, not only did expansion become intractable, but so too did exiting to different avenues of policymaking. For example, policymakers' efforts in 1974 to exit to alternative paths on behalf of universal coverage were already difficult, because they were extremely expensive and threatened a number of private interests that had a stake in the system as it existed. But organized labor flatly refused to compromise its position of advocating pure social insurance expansion (thereby blocking any exit). Its ideological commitment to a Social Security style health insurance plan was accompanied by practical economic interests: Labor insisted on a health insurance program similar to Social Security—one that was universal, comprehensive, and, most important, protected from inflation: three characteristics that their private, collectively bargained plans lacked.[8] Even liberal advocates of universal coverage in Congress, such as Senator Ted Kennedy, concluded that exhorting organized labor to pursue a compromise plan was basically a dialogue with the deaf (see chapter 6). Gambling that the 1974 elections would vindicate its position that the public path was still open to expansion, labor lost. The onset of recession in late 1974 demonstrated that the public path was, in fact, closed.

Soon after this window of opportunity for change closed in 1974, OASDI's and Medicare's costs exploded. Policymakers had to focus on trying to control the two programs' expenditures through major program rationalization (Medicare's Prospective Payment System in 1983, and OASDI's bailouts in 1977 and 1983). When President Clinton chose to take advantage of the next incident of rising public interest in comprehensive health care reform in the early 1990s, the accumulated costs of inherited programs made any new public commitments to the uninsured extraordinarily expensive.

The Blessing and Curse of Medicare

This is essentially the story of universal health coverage first being subordinated to old age insurance, repeatedly blocked by organized medicine, and then crowded out by deeply entrenched, vested interests and the astronomical growth of Social Security's and Medicare's costs. It affirms Theodore Marmor and Andrew Dunham's assertion that health care policy in the United States evolved in such a clientele-oriented manner that it rendered comprehensive change impossible.[9] Policymakers' passage of Medicare was a seminal event in health care policy, as well as a major political victory for their strategy of incrementalism. According to Marmor and Jerry Mashaw, though, Medicare was only a first step:

> The incrementalist strategy assumed that [Medicare] was a first step in benefits and that more would follow under the usual pattern of Social Security financing. Supporters thought of Medicare as national health insurance for a population group, universally covering retirees and, later, the disabled. Likewise, proponents presumed that eligibility would be gradually expanded. Eventually,

they believed, Medicare would take in most, if not all, of the population, with the first extension perhaps being made to children and pregnant women. The kind of full inclusion envisaged here meant workers and their families, not literally every citizen or person in the land. But there was no mistaking the Medicare strategists' aspiration toward ever broader coverage. . . .

The form adopted for Medicare—Social Security financing and eligibility for hospital care and premiums, plus general revenues for physician expenses—had a political explanation, not a consistent social insurance rationale. . . .

Viewed as a first step, of course, the Medicare strategy made sense.[10]

Nevertheless, Medicare also permanently fragmented the nation's health care system. It cemented the pattern of having different programs—along public and private paths—collectively meet the majority of the population's need for medical care. As a result, the United States' health care system evolved into a highly complex weave of different programs and policies replete with politically powerful and entrenched vested interests: private, tax-subsidized, employer-provided health insurance for workers; Medicare for the elderly; Medicaid for the poor; the Veterans Administration for veterans; and nothing for the roughly 40 million uncovered individuals who fall in between.

So any effort to achieve universal coverage through comprehensive change has been overwhelmed with reconciling new proposals with old programs and commitments. Repeated success with incremental expansion led to a social insurance system that could no longer afford additional commitments, but it also hindered the new financial arrangements required in any reform designed to attain universal coverage, such as Clinton's 1993-94 Health Security Act.

There is some evidence that incrementalism is not totally defunct. Rather, policymakers may have, ironically, switched the strategy's path to that of state-administered welfare (e.g., the State Children's Health Insurance Program or SCHIP).[11] But it is too early yet to know if a program such as SCHIP is truly representative of a major new approach to achieving universal coverage through "welfare" incrementalism.

Another welfare program for medical care, Medicaid, was able to serve as a platform upon which policymakers could incrementally expand to the benefit of pregnant women and children. But policymakers could never expand enough to reach universal coverage, largely because Congress has consistently maintained its means-tested requirements below the level necessary for insuring those without private health coverage. Thus, many individuals are too poor for private health insurance but too rich for public health insurance. In addition, Medicaid's range has been expanded—at the expense of its scope—to cover nonuniversal coverage issues as nursing home care for a large proportion of the nation's senior citizens.[12]

Are We Approaching the Next Critical Juncture?

Two trends that began in the late 1990s suggest that the U.S. health care system may be approaching another critical juncture. First, despite the decade's record economic expansion, Marie Gottschalk notes, "an average of a million Americans a year have either lost their health insurance or failed to obtain insurance for which they became eligible."[13] Second, after falling in the early 1990s (see figure 7.5) and holding steady during the mid-1990s, health insurance premiums have increased significantly since 1997 (figure 8.1). These trends suggest that although managed care emerged in the 1990s as the dominant private paradigm, its savings were limited to the short term. Moreover, managed care has done nothing to address the problem of the uninsured, because it is not designed to.

Figure 8.1
Rate of Increase in Health Insurance Premiums, 1994-2000

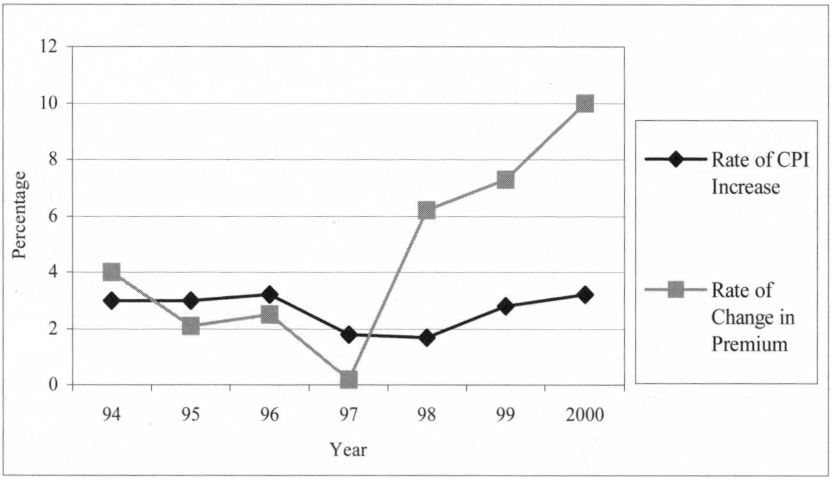

Source: Annual Change in CPI from the U.S. Dept. of Labor, Bureau of Labor Statistics: Mercer-Higgins Survey of Employers Sponsored Health Plans, 1999; and NHCH Projections. See also, Joel E. Miller, "Déjà vu All Over Again," National Coalition on Health Care (Washington, D.C.: May 2000), ii, 1.

By the end of the Clinton administration, the same two trends that made health care reform so salient in the very early 1990s returned. "The rising cost of health insurance and the growing number of the uninsured are interconnected," argues Joel Miller. "They will continue to affect each other, because the growing number of uninsured patients means that providers will try to pass on those costs to employers and employees who are able to pay. The result will be even higher premium increases, which in turn cause more people to become uninsured. These problems will not self-correct."[14] The logical conclusion is that policymakers will have to correct them. But the findings of this research reveal how enormously difficult it is for reformers to enact large-scale changes to the American health care system.

Living with Political Consequences

The critical junctures that occur in nations ordinarily garner the bulk of political scientists' attention. This is logical, because major change (such as Social Security's passage in 1935) is both fascinating and hugely determinative of what comes thereafter. Instances of fundamental change or revolutionary reform in well-institutionalized political systems attract the most attention precisely because they are so rare.[15]

But equally significant are the patterns that critical junctures set in motion, which over time become distinct paths of policymaking. These paths frequently generate increasing returns that make them continually more attractive for individuals and organizations who, in turn, adjust their behavior in a way that strongly reinforces the paths to which they are adjusting. This reinforcing phenomenon produces an equilibrium: Social needs—such as medical care and supplemental retirement income—gradually conform to dominant modes of provision (be they private or public).

This analysis has demonstrated that in those programs and patterns subject to an unusually high degree of increasing returns, such as OASDI and to a slightly lesser extent employer-provided health insurance, three factors play prominent roles:

> A. *Contingency*. Relatively small events, if occurring at the right moment, can have large and enduring consequences. Accidents can matter.

> B. *Timing and sequencing* become crucial. In increasing returns processes, when an event occurs may be just as important as what occurs. Because early parts of a sequence matter much more than later parts, an event that happens "too late" may have no impact, though it might have been of great consequence if the timing had been different.

> C. *Inertia*. Once an increasing returns process has been established, social actors will face strong pressures to adapt, and these adaptations will generally lead to a single equilibrium. This equilibrium will in turn be strongly resistant to change. Once down the path, inertia will be prevalent.[16]

History reveals that programmatic additions such as disability insurance and Medicare—made possible only by Social Security—came at a future cost. Together with uncharacteristically large OASDI benefit increases between 1966 and 1972, these programmatic additions grew so expensive that they contributed to the blocking of any more expansion. And the new constituencies they produced became opposed to exiting to new policy paths for achieving universal coverage because doing so threatened the arrangements and benefits to which they had become accustomed. Just as increasing returns were effective in enlarging Social Security's policy commitments prior to 1972, decreasing returns became effective in precluding new social insurance commitments after 1972.

This analysis might leave advocates of universal coverage, liberal and conservative alike, with a sense of discouragement. The conclusion could be that the future is rigidly dictated by decisions in the past that cannot be readdressed, much less changed. This would be overstating the case and ignoring how the entire analysis began—with a critical juncture in 1935 (in the form of Social Security) that few if any could ever have foreseen at the time. As previously noted, critical junctures are rare, but they do occur and are ordinarily in response to acute, but unmet social needs. So there is hope.

Notes

1. Social Security did incorporate a national health insurance scheme, Medicare, but it was an incomplete one.

2. Their efforts have been largely successful, if success is defined by avoiding financial default and bankruptcy. Neither OASDI nor Medicare has experienced this fate, and both are firmly institutionalized. True, the strategy of incremental expansion is virtually defunct, but any actual exiting to alternative forms of old age provision (income and health insurance) has been noticeable for its absence. Privatization in some measure has been seriously discussed, but to date nothing material has come from this discussion. If Medicare and OASDI's histories suggest anything about the future possibility of exiting to alternative policy paths, it is that only impending financial calamity (as in 1977 and 1983) can make dramatic change possible. But even the dramatic change that has occurred has only adjusted the programs' reimbursement and financing features. Neither in 1977 nor in 1983 did policymakers actually exit to an alternative path for either program.

3. See nn. 14-16, ch. 1.

4. Paul David, "Clio and the Economics of QWERTY," *American Economic Review* 75 (May 1985): 335.

5. Since 1965, many individuals past age sixty-five and the poor have come to rely on the public programs of Medicare and Medicaid, respectively.

6. Robert H. Bates et al., *Analytic Narratives* (Princeton, N.J.: Princeton University Press, 1998), 8.

7. This experience of policymakers using incrementalism at the margins of society's institutional landscape to affect policy change conforms to Douglass C. North's theory of institutional change. See Douglass C. North, *Institutions, Institutional Change, and Economic Performance* (Cambridge: Cambridge University Press, 1990), 7-8. See also, Paul Pierson, "Increasing Returns, Path Dependence, and the Study of Politics," Program for the Study of Germany and Europe, Working Paper Series 7.7 (Center for European Studies, Harvard University, September 1, 1997), 12.

8. With the health insurance component of union contracts unable to keep pace with rising prices, workers' out-of-pocket costs continued to rise. For more information, see "The Case for National Health Insurance," *AFL-CIO American Federationist* (January 1970): 9-10. For full quote of the AFL-CIO's president, George Meany, explaining why labor wanted a pure Social Security-style national health insurance plan, see ch. 6.

9. Theodore R. Marmor and Andrew B. Dunham, "Federal Policy and Health," in *Nationalizing Government: Public Policies in America*, ed. T. Lowi and A. Stone (London: Sage Publications, 1978), 267: "United States financing programs continue to be a

series of discrete programs aimed at specific clientele." Marmor and Dunham's assertion in 1978 is only truer today.

10. Theodore R. Marmor and Jerry L. Mashaw, "The Case for Social Insurance," in *The New Majority*, ed. S. B. Greenberg and Theda Skocpol (New Haven, Conn.: Yale University Press, 1997), 96-97.

11. See Marsha Gold, "Markets and Medicaid," in *Healthy Markets? The New Competition in Medical Care*, ed. Mark E. Peterson (Durham, N.C.: Duke University Press, 1998), 285; and Daniel Palazzolo, *Done Deal? The Politics of the 1997 Budget Agreement* (New York: Chatham House, 1999), 130-31, 136-37, 184-85.

12. See Joshua Wiener, "Reducing Medicaid Spending on Long-Term Care," 1999, Urban Institute, <www.urban.org/periodcl/26_2/prr26_2e.htm> (8 August 1999); Peter J. Ferrara, "Long-Term Care: Why a New Entitlement Program Would Be Wrong," 1990, Cato Institute, <www.cato.org/pubs/pas/pa-144.html> (8 August 1999).

13. Marie Gottschalk, *The Shadow Welfare State: Labor, Business, and the Politics of Health Care in the United States* (Ithaca, N.Y.: Cornell University Press, 2000), 4. See also, Joel E. Miller, "Déjà vu All Over Again: The Soaring Cost of Private Health Insurance and Its Impact on Consumers and Employers," *National Coalition on Health Care* (Washington, D.C.: May 2000).

14. Miller, "Déjà All Over Again," 22.

15. Pierson, "Increasing Returns, Path Dependence, and the Study of Politics," Working Paper Series 7.7, 30.

16. Pierson, "Increasing Returns, Path Dependence, and the Study of Politics," Working Paper Series 7.7, 31.

EPILOGUE, 2004

One of my administration's top priorities is high quality, affordable health care for all Americans.

—President George W. Bush
State of the Union Address, January 2003

I think we're standing on the edge of a cliff . . . I've become more convinced as time goes by that our health care system is fundamentally broken and needs major surgery; it's collapsing around us.

—U.S. Senator John Breaux
March 2003

But thou, O Lord, how long?

—King David
Psalm 6:3

Another health care crisis has emerged in the United States. It was inevitable. As the previous chapters illustrate, the patchwork quilt of individual government programs and private insurance arrangements that collectively make up the U.S. health care system has numerous structural contradictions, economic inefficiencies, and coverage gaps for millions of Americans. It's no wonder that studying our country's health care system often produces the same reaction one has after studying Italian politics and finance: How does such a Byzantine, sometimes corrupt, and fundamentally illogical structure such as this survive, much less thrive in various areas? It reminds one of the Leaning Tower of Pisa. One marvels at its existence and wonders how much longer it can remain standing. It appears to defy the law of gravity, but everyone talks about it only being a matter of time before the structure comes crumbling down. The mystery is that nobody knows or ever can know exactly when it will happen. Similarly, how many uninsured individuals, medically impoverished patients, frustrated physicians, burnt-out nurses, and cash-strapped businesses need to exist before a critical mass finally materializes that flushes out the formidable political obstacles to some form of universal coverage in the U.S.? One guess is as good as another. But what is clear is that our country's health care system is experiencing a number of major interrelated problems.

Is Our Patchwork Health Care System Unraveling?

Ten years after President Clinton's ambitious attempt at comprehensive health care reform died so ignominiously, the same problems—only worse—have returned and some new ones have appeared. The following is a brief overview of just some of the leading ills plaguing many Americans and, more generally, our nation's health care system.

After declining modestly in 1999 and 2000, at the height of the country's economic boom, the number of uninsured Americans rose to 45 million (or 15.6 percent of the population in 2003).[1] These figures have likely increased since then. The lack of health insurance coverage has become as much a "working class" and "middle class" phenomenon as it is a "poor" one. Roughly a third of all Americans earning between $25,000 and $75,000 (or 21,500,000 individuals) are uninsured.[2] More than 75 percent of the uninsured work full-time and about a third earn more than $50,000.[3] If you include individuals who have experienced a temporary lack of coverage, the number of Americans without health insurance at some point during the last two years rose to 75 million in 2002, which is nearly one third of all Americans younger than 65.[4] Even the affluent are not immune. The number of uninsured people with household incomes of $75,000 or more rose to 7.3 million in 2002, an increase of 633,000 from the year before.[5]

Not only are there millions of Americans without insurance, the costs for those who do have it are increasing rapidly. Unlike a decade ago, when health care costs and insurance premiums were decreasing, they have been steadily rising and more than the general rate of inflation since 1998. Total national spending on health care grew 8.6 percent in 2002, marking the biggest one-year increase since 1993.[6] Employers' health insurance premiums rose by an average of almost 14 percent in 2003—more than anticipated and the largest increase since 1990.[7] Small companies of less than ten employees have seen their insurance premiums rise, provided they can still afford them, by as much as 20 percent or more per year since 2001.[8] And the future does not look better. "The number of uninsured will continue to grow as long as health insurance premiums rise more rapidly than earnings, as they have for a decade," notes Drew E. Altman, president of the Kaiser Family Foundation, which tracks health coverage trends. "Losing health benefits is becoming a middle-class issue. If it had not been for expansions in the child health program and Medicaid, we would have 10 million more uninsured."[9]

One particularly alarming consequence of these worsening trends is that health care related problems are one of the leading causes of personal bankruptcy in the United States. Upwards of 600,000 individual cases in 1999, or nearly 50 percent of the total number of non-business bankruptcy filings, were traceable to one or more of these problems: lack of health insurance, insufficient health insurance, and/or substantial medical bills.[10] Given the recession and sluggish economic growth that have occurred since then, it is certain that these figures have only worsened.

The government's two primary health insurance programs—Medicare for the elderly and disabled and Medicaid for the poor—are experiencing considerable financial strain. As they face their worst fiscal crises in more than fifty years, states are cutting Medicaid benefits and eligibility at the same time that a sputtering economy has boosted demand for the program.[11] Meanwhile, Medicare has suffered from two high-profile problems: a failed experiment with enrolling beneficiaries in private managed care plans (Medicare+Choice), and an inability to find a fiscally responsible way to add prescription drug coverage to the program. In March 2004—four months after President Bush signed the new Medicare Prescription Drug, Improvement and Modernization Act into law on December 8, 2003—a scandal erupted over the disclosure that Medicare's chief actuary had originally estimated the cost of the new drug plan to be closer to $550 billion over 10 years rather than the $400 billion figure that lawmakers were led to believe and which they used in their political deliberations.[12]

Not only are many of the poor and elderly often inadequately served by our health care system, so too are many children. Despite the progress achieved by SCHIP (the State Children's Health Insurance Program) since 1997, 8.5 million or 12 percent of all youngsters are still uninsured.[13] What is worse, a combination of factors is expected to reduce enrollment in SCHIP and *increase* the number of uninsured children by 900,000 by 2007.[14] These factors include: pending reductions in federal SCHIP funding, the expected reversion of previously allocated federal SCHIP funds to the U.S. Treasury, and growing state budget crises.

The new health care crisis is affecting doctors as much as patients. Medical malpractice insurance has become an enormous problem for specific specialties: obstetricians, neurosurgeons, radiologists, and emergency room physicians in particular. Many women in Arizona, for instance, now have to drive an hour or more to reach a hospital with a delivery room; the entire state of West Virginia has at times been without the services of a neurosurgeon; and many doctors in West Virginia, New Jersey, Pennsylvania, Florida, Mississippi, Illinois, Texas and Missouri have held or threatened to hold work stoppages.[15] The AMA estimates that medical liability insurance has reached crisis proportions in 18 states and is nearing crisis proportions in 26 other states.[16] Younger physicians in training have noticed this crisis, along with other problems in our health care system. A quarter of final-year medical students polled said they would not study medicine if they could start their education over again.[17]

How has it all come to this? The following sections address each of these problems in greater depth and show how they are often interconnected. Included in this epilogue is a reexamination of President Clinton's epic failure at health care reform based largely on interviews with several key policymakers and staff of that time. Some of those interviewed have only recently granted interviews about why and how everything came to naught in 1993-94. The epilogue concludes with a brief overview of the leading proposals for solving the problem of the uninsured that have recently emerged. If they seem similar to previous proposals dating back to the early 1970s, it is because they are: hauntingly so. As Yogi Berra once said, "It seems like déjà vu all over again."

Health Insurance and the Increasing Numbers of Those Without It

It is hard to grasp the magnitude of the number of uninsured, as Ronald F. Pollack, executive director of Families USA, has observed. It exceeds the aggregate population of 24 states. Nevertheless, in the late 1990s the prospects for reaching universal coverage seemed to be slightly improving. From 1994 to 2000, a period of extraordinary economic prosperity, the rate of the uninsured at least remained steady and even fell a little in 1999 and 2000. This improvement appeared to be the result of two things: an expansion in employer-provided coverage and a decrease in the number of previously uninsured children (thanks to the introduction of SCHIP and changes to Medicaid). This was initially encouraging. The private sector looked as if it was more than matching the public sector's increased generosity (Medicaid and SCHIP in particular).[18]

As it turns out, the primary reason for the overall increase in health insurance coverage during this period (1994-2000) was a large contingent of Americans who moved up the income-ladder. During this period, employers were not beset with a spasmodic burst of generosity as much as a "tight labor market allowed people to take jobs with higher earnings and a higher likelihood of employer coverage."[19] Employers had to either pay higher salaries and provide health insurance during this period or lose potential employees to their competitors. That all changed beginning in 2001, when the U.S. economy went into recession and 1.4 million Americans lost their health insurance coverage.[20]

The most striking lesson from the mid to late 1990s is that prosperity does not solve the problem of the uninsured. The country experienced the longest stretch of uninterrupted economic growth (120 months from March 1991 to March 2001) ever recorded, budget surpluses returned after thirty years of continuous and rising deficits, and unemployment levels hit lows not seen since the 1960s. Yet the rate of the uninsured barely budged. The tremendous economic wave of the 1990s that raised just about every "boat" had little to no effect on the 15 percent of Americans without health insurance.

There are three main reasons for the erosion of private health coverage that began in 2001.[21] First, unemployment increased. The unemployment rate averaged 4.8 percent at the beginning of 2001, 5.9 percent in 2002, and 6.4 percent by the summer of 2003. Because the majority of American workers and their dependents receive health insurance coverage from their employers, increasing unemployment leads directly to greater numbers of uninsured people.

Second, fewer businesses are offering health coverage.[22] A survey by the Kaiser Family Foundation found that premiums for employer-provided insurance have climbed an average of 12.7 percent since 2001. Consequently, more small and medium-size companies can no longer afford to offer coverage. While 67 percent of companies with fewer than 200 employees offered health benefits to their workers in 2000, only 61 percent did so in 2002.[23]

Finally, job-based coverage is becoming too expensive for many workers. Employers of all sizes are passing on more of their increasing health care costs to their workers and retirees in the form of larger co-payments, deductibles, and monthly premiums (particularly for workers' dependents).[24] Kate Sullivan, director of health policy at the United States Chamber of Commerce, noted that many employers continue to subsidize insurance for workers, but have reduced subsidies for dependents. She adds, "A lot of insurers are dropping out of the small-group market, and customers are balking at what they have to pay."[25]

Much of the recent increase in health care costs and insurance premiums can be attributed to the demise of managed care (except for the Medicaid and SCHIP populations) and the reversion to fee-for-service payment. Many of the administrative rules and procedures that made managed care so successful in temporarily containing costs were despised by both patients and medical providers. Hence, over time most were either legislated or litigated out of existence. Employers' transition to managed care effectively controlled costs for a period in the 1990s, largely because they were able to squeeze payments to physicians and hospitals. In short, there was a lot of "fat" in the health care system that could easily be eliminated through annual, competitive negotiations between insurers (or managed care organizations) and medical providers. After much of the "fat" was removed, however, these cost cutting strategies proved to be short-lived and unsustainable.

In time, Alain Enthoven notes, "traditional, restrictive managed care has broken down under an onslaught of attacks from attorneys, politicians, patients, and providers. Consequently, we are now back to runaway health care inflation, with annual premium increases of 15 to 20 percent or more in some areas."[26] Many physicians are still discouraged to the point of retiring early or switching careers altogether. Meanwhile, health maintenance organizations (HMOs) remain under attack. Patients resent administrative restrictions to their receiving medical care just as much as (if not more than) providers resent restrictions to their providing it. Thus, many employers have been moving away from the rigid, cost-conscious managed care plans to more lightly managed preferred provider models (PPOs) and, in some cases, even reverting entirely to traditional fee-for-service insurance arrangements.[27]

Although the older version of managed care has died a protracted death, one specific event proved symbolic of its burial. Aetna, one of the nation's biggest health insurers, settled a long-running lawsuit with almost all of the approximately 700,000 practicing physicians in the country in late May 2003. Aetna agreed to pay a $100 million fine (to the doctors), establish a foundation for the improvement of health care (to the tune of $20 million), and to pay the doctors' lawyers up to $50 million for their work on the case. The suit alleged that Aetna unlawfully interfered with physicians' medical and billing decisions. In settling the case, Aetna gave up on the classic form of managed care, which was originally designed around so-called gatekeepers: Aetna administrators "who approved or denied coverage for treatments, often for reasons that were obscure both to doctors and patients."[28] The settlement was a victory for physicians and signaled the end of restrictive managed care. Unfortunately, this means that health care costs and rates of the uninsured are likely to increase.[29]

Who are the uninsured? Compared to the general population, the uninsured tend to be younger and have somewhat lower incomes and less education; they are more likely to be members of minority groups, and to work in service industries and for smaller companies (figures E-1, E-2).[30] The uninsured population is a dynamic group: individuals often have insurance one year and don't have it the next. People move in and out of coverage depending on their employment status, marital status, income, age, and numerous other factors. The changing nature of the uninsured makes it extremely difficult to fashion a single policy or program to address the problem.

Figure E-1
People without Health Insurance, 2002

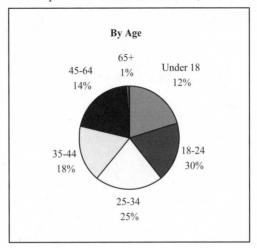

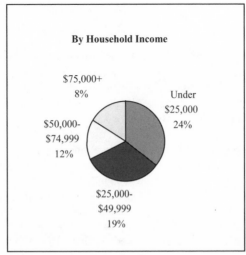

Source: U.S. Census Bureau, 2003

Figure E-2
People without Health Insurance, 2002

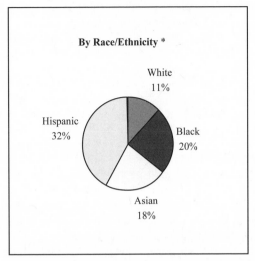

By Race/Ethnicity *

White
11%

Hispanic
32%

Black
20%

Asian
18%

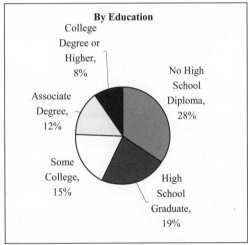

By Education

College
Degree or
Higher,
8%

No High
School
Diploma,
28%

Associate
Degree,
12%

Some
College,
15%

High
School
Graduate,
19%

Source: U.S. Census Bureau, 2003
* Hispanics may be of any race, so figures are rounded.

A related concern is the growing number of working Americans who are classified as "covered" by health insurance who really have little to no coverage at all. An estimated 750,000 employees and their dependents have what are known as "limited benefit" plans. The premiums are low (roughly $7 per week), but they pay only a maximum of $1,000 a year in medical bills—so little that "some question whether it amounts to health insurance at all," acknowledged the *Wall Street Journal*. "Some in the insurance industry have a hard time taking this coverage seriously. A gathering of 300 insurance agents in Las Vegas erupted into laughter last summer when an insurance-company executive explained a limited-benefit plan offered by Star Human Resources."[31] Unfortunately, these policies are among the fastest-growing health insurance offerings in the workplace. Enrollment in the plans has grown about 20 percent in the past two years alone. They are especially popular among low-wage employees at Wal-Mart, McDonalds, and Lowe's Company.[32] Granted, some measure of health coverage is better than none. But these policies are dangerously close to nothing. And what is perhaps most worrying is that more employers are likely to drop their traditional health benefits for these limited benefit plans. As the cost to employers of providing comprehensive health benefits has risen almost 60% in the past five years—to an average of about $5,700 per employee per year— more service employers might find it irresistible to just offer limited benefit plans that would not cover one full day in the hospital or an MRI.[*]

Losing health insurance has always registered as a leading fear among people of all income levels, because it is well known that a prolonged illness or medical emergency can—more than perhaps any other unpredictable calamity— destroy a family's or an individual's financial security. If only it were a matter, then, of attaining universal coverage. What was so striking about the widely read April 2000 report by Elizabeth Warren, Teresa Sullivan and Melissa Jacoby, "Medical Problems and Bankruptcy Filings," was that of the 596,198 families that filed for bankruptcy in 1999 due at least in part to a "medical reason," about 80 percent of them had health coverage.[33]

The authors also found that nearly half of all bankruptcies involved a medical problem, and certain groups—particularly women heads of households and the elderly—were even more likely to report a health-related bankruptcy. The fact that 80 percent of those who declared bankruptcy had some form of coverage indicates that basic health insurance often does not protect families from financial disaster when they suffer serious medical problems. Families may be left with medical bills that exhaust their health insurance coverage, or "they may discover that the income effects, such as lost time from work or a shift to less physically demanding work, impose a financial hardship on a family that basic medical insurance simply does not cover."[34]

Revisiting the issue in 2002, Professor Warren indicated that families filing for bankruptcy represented a cross-section of America. For instance, she discovered that their educations were slightly better than the U.S. average. More than half were homeowners, and their occupations were typical of the range of occupations in the U.S. job market. By most criteria, about 90 percent of the

---

[*] If, for whatever reason, you find yourself worrying about how chief executives have weathered the efforts by companies to pare or eliminate their most expensive benefit, medical insurance, don't. Roughly one in eight U.S. companies offers what are known as "executive medical-expense reimbursement plans." These plans pay for chief executives' deductibles, co-payments, and other out-of-pocket medical expenses—in some cases even as the same companies are cutting back on basic medical coverage for their rank-and-file workers. See Carol Hymowitz and Joann S. Lublin, "Benefits: I'll Have What He's Having," *Wall Street Journal*, May 20, 2003, B1.

debtors in bankruptcy would be classified as solidly middle-class; however, two out of three lost a job at some point shortly before filing, and nearly half had medical problems.[35]

Invariably, growing numbers of under- and uninsured Americans increase the pressure on the country's public health insurance programs (Medicaid, SCHIP, and Medicare). These programs are already facing serious funding and demographic problems. So it is worth investigating the extent to which they can assume a much greater responsibility for providing health care to individuals who used to have private coverage.

We turn first to Medicaid, the program most people view as the joint federal-state health insurance program for poor women and their children. In actuality, Medicaid is an immense and remarkably flexible program that both state and federal policymakers have continually modified over the past decade and a half to address an array of society's unmet health care needs, including those of the indigent elderly and disabled. In the process, the program relieves the suffering of millions of people who fall through the numerous holes in our country's health care system.

Medicaid: The Ugly, Unloved "Workhorse" of the U.S. Health Care System

This book is an excellent example, unfortunately, of how Medicaid has been largely ignored—relative to Medicare—and labeled a topic for poverty studies and welfare policy. Because much of this book's analysis focuses on Medicare as a seminal achievement in social insurance and its evolution into a major roadblock to universal coverage, Medicaid receives only passing attention. This partly reflects the fact that when Medicaid was enacted in 1965, it was considered "a legislative afterthought to Medicare."[36] Fortunately, this epilogue provides an opportunity to reexamine a program that, unlike Medicare, bears little resemblance to its original 1966 structure and, according to 2002 data, has surpassed Medicare in numbers of beneficiaries (51 million to Medicare's 41 million) while almost equaling it in terms of total spending (roughly $250 billion).[37]

As the nation's largest health insurance program, Medicaid insures 20 percent of the nation's children and, surprisingly, pays for more than one in every three childbirths.[38] Although the program's original focus was on poor mothers who received welfare and their children, it has expanded into something of a subsidiary program to Medicare for impoverished senior citizens and the disabled. Medicaid now provides for the care that two-thirds of the nation's nursing home residents receive. It also helps more than 6 million low-income Medicare beneficiaries pay their monthly Medicare Part B premiums and prescription drug costs.[39] Medicaid finances the bulk of the care provided to AIDS patients, half of all states' mental health services, and one-sixth of the nation's pharmaceutical drug expenses. The program even provides the financial glue that holds together the nation's "safety net" institutions: most teaching hospitals, community and migrant health centers, psychiatric hospitals, and community-based facilities which treat persons with mental disorders. These institutions are critical in a nation where, at any given point in time, almost 1 in every 6 individuals does not have the means to pay for substantial medical bills.[40]

As the program "called upon to solve all manner of health-related problems that no other institution or sector of the economy is willing to address," Alan Weil explains, Medicaid is still

> a program loved by few, denigrated by many, and misunderstood by most. It is at least three different programs in one:
>
> (1) A source of traditional insurance coverage for poor children and some of their parents;
>
> (2) A payer for a complex range of acute and long-term care services for the frail elderly and people with physical disabilities and mental illness, many of whom were once middle class; and
>
> (3) A source of wraparound coverage for low-income elders on Medicare.[41]

Medicaid is frequently ignored, if not disdained, by many Americans because it is a "poor people's program." Like any form of means-tested public assistance, beneficiaries have not earned their way into Medicaid (like Medicare and Social Security). Yet this has allowed policymakers to modify the program's eligibility and benefits over time in response to various unmet health care needs. Responsibility for financing Medicaid is split between the states and the federal government, which pays between 50 and 77 percent depending on each state's per capita income (wealthier states pay closer to 50 percent, poorer states closer to 23 percent). Last year the federal government paid for 57 percent of the program's total cost (approximately $259 billion).[42]

What surprises many people about Medicaid is the extent to which the program, initially intended for poor single mothers and their children, has expanded to serve as a "safety net" for the elderly and disabled. Women and children represent about 75 percent of the program's enrollment, but only 30 percent of its spending (figure E-3). Able-bodied, childless adults are not eligible for Medicaid regardless of their income level. Most of the program's expenditures go to cover the elderly and disabled who, as a group, are in poorer health compared to single women and children. The single largest category of Medicaid spending is nursing home care. Moreover, "while almost all nursing facility, ICF-MR (intermediate care facilities for the mentally retarded), and home health spending is on behalf of the elderly and disabled," observes Weil, "this group also accounts for 85 percent of prescription drug costs, more than half of inpatient and outpatient hospital spending, and nearly half of physician services."[43]

Medicaid's growing role as a safety net for these two expensive and growing populations—the disabled and indigent elderly—has prevented it from becoming an even broader "safety net" for the uninsured. This dilemma is exacerbated by the fact that the states, facing their worst fiscal shortfalls in decades, are currently looking for ways to restrain their second most expensive program's costs (after K-12 education), not expand its eligibility.[44]

Figure E-3
Medicaid Enrollment and Spending, by Eligibility Group, 2002

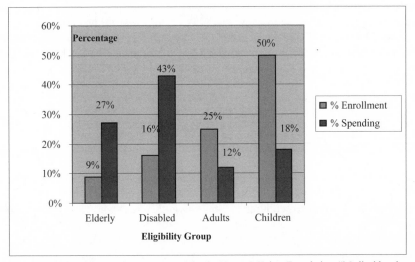

Source: Urban Institute estimates prepared for the Henry J. Kaiser Foundation, "Medicaid and the Uninsured: The Medicaid Program at a Glance" (Washington: Kaiser Commission on Medicaid and the Uninsured, January 2004).

What is perhaps most unfortunate about Medicaid's growing status as a "hole-patcher" for Medicare is that, irony of ironies, the past two decades have shown the former to be a much more promising vehicle for reaching universal coverage than the latter. Health reformers have traditionally envisioned it the other way around, with Medicare being the vehicle for reaching the goal. But as Lawrence Brown and Michael Sparer point out, Medicare's benefits and beneficiaries have not changed much since the program's passage. Medicaid, on the other hand, has maintained its relatively extensive benefits in the face of economic uncertainty while significantly expanding its eligibility criteria. Moreover, although Medicare has attractive universal coverage for all senior citizens and the disabled, it has forgone the flexibility states have enjoyed with Medicaid in crafting creative structural solutions and implementing reforms such as managed care.[45]

The best example of Medicaid's ability to broaden the level of health insurance coverage—in a way that Medicare never has—is SCHIP (the State Children's Health Insurance Program). SCHIP constitutes the nation's single biggest expansion of public health insurance eligibility since Medicare and Medicaid's passage in 1965. Enacted in the Balanced Budget Act of 1997, the program follows the Medicaid model: federal matching funds for programs in which states have wide discretion. SCHIP also allows states to reach the program's target, uninsured children who do not qualify for Medicaid, by making SCHIP an addition to their Medicaid programs.[46]

SCHIP is something of the "Kiddiecare" program that social insurance enthusiasts always envisioned adding to Medicare, but which never could be done because of Medicare's cost explosion.[47] Consequently, the strategy of incrementalism that stalled in the 1970s was transferred to the welfare path of Medicaid, which policymakers (notably Representative Henry Waxman, D-CA) have cleverly and discreetly expanded by way of the annual budget process. Yet SCHIP, like Medicaid upon which it is modeled, also illustrates the limits and disadvantages of expanding health insurance incrementally via the welfare model. Because, unlike social insurance, what the government giveth in the form of public assistance, it can also taketh away (figure E-4).

SCHIP: Covering the Children of Uninsured, Working Parents

As the largest expansion of eligibility for government health insurance since Medicare and Medicaid in 1965, policymakers created SCHIP in 1997 to reduce the number of uninsured children (10 million at the time) who were not covered by Medicaid.[48] The program, Title XXI of the Social Security Act, was a response to a growing economic phenomenon in our country: a family's household income is too low to afford private health insurance but too high to qualify for existing public health insurance.

Currently, about 70 percent of uninsured children live in a household whose total income is more than $15,670—the 2004 poverty line for a family of three and the maximum level of income for Medicaid eligibility—but less than $31,340 (200 percent above the poverty line).[49] The vast majority of uninsured children have a parent who works full-time (75 percent) or at least part-time (10 percent).[50] These families, however, are either not offered health insurance by their employers or they cannot afford to purchase it.[51]

SCHIP resembles Medicaid's structure in that the program is jointly financed. The federal government's share ranges from 65 to 84 percent, depending on each state's portion of the nation's total number of uninsured children. The states were given a great deal of discretion in constructing their SCHIP programs, and encouragement to be generous with their eligibility criteria. States could create a new program, expand their Medicaid program to include children eligible under SCHIP, or devise a combination of both. By 2000, every state and U.S. territory had a SCHIP program in place. Currently, 21 states and territories are operating Medicaid expansion programs, 16 have separate SCHIP programs, and 19 are operating combination Medicaid/SCHIP programs.[52] Similar to Medicaid, most state SCHIP plans rely on—and are the last bastions of—traditional, restrictive managed care to control their costs.[53]

The states were initially excited about insuring more children, particularly as the robust economy of the late 1990s provided them with surplus funds that were more than matched by the federal government. States took great pride in the new opportunity to develop their SCHIP programs and to reach out to low-income families. According to Jennifer Ryan, they set up marketing campaigns, held outreach events featuring their governors, and came up with catchy names—such as Healthy Kids, Peach Care, and Hoosier Healthwise—for their new SCHIP programs. Behind the scenes, states also simplified their programs to make them more user-friendly. According to Ryan, "they shortened applications, encouraged families to apply by mail instead of making them come to a welfare office, and removed some of the tedious and burdensome eligibility verification requirements. The federal government did its part to raise awareness of the program. President Clinton and other members of the administration hosted many SCHIP events, including the launch of a nationwide outreach campaign, Insure Kids Now, that includes a toll-free number and Web site where families can call and be linked directly with enrollment information for SCHIP in their state."[54] As figure E-4 shows, the result of these initial efforts has been encouraging. Enrollment has risen steadily from about 1 million children in 1998 to 5.3 million by 2002.

In addition to reaching millions of uninsured children, the most promising SCHIP-related development was the way in which the program made universal coverage more attainable. This new possibility came by way of a number of states expanding their SCHIP coverage to include the uninsured parents of eligible children. The theory has been that making the program more generous and available to parents would help states reach more eligible children. Studies of the first four states to cover parents of children enrolled in SCHIP—New Jersey, Minnesota, Rhode Island, and Wisconsin—found that the experiment worked exceedingly well in increasing the numbers of enrolled children and, concurrently, reducing the state's overall rate of uninsured individuals by also insuring more uncovered adults.[55]

But while Medicaid and SCHIP have played innovative roles in keeping millions of working families from bankruptcy, crushing medical debt, and/or ill health, their structure shows the inherent limits of welfare programs that are means-tested and financed by general revenues. First, less than 50 percent of the children covered by SCHIP appear to be retained by the program when their eligibility is redetermined each year.[56] This is partly explained by the parents of eligible children either becoming poorer and, thus, qualifying for Medicaid or wealthier and, thus, ineligible for either program. Neither of these explanations for a child being dropped from the SCHIP program is a reason for concern because they are (hopefully) still covered. However, in some states the retention rate is as low as 26 percent and change to parents' income only explains a portion of this very low number. Many of these "lost" children appear to be the result of parents who are confused about the rules and procedures they are to follow to keep their children's coverage up to date.[57] It is exceedingly discouraging to realize that there are still millions of children without access to regular medical care and insurance protection solely due to bureaucratic misunderstandings or their parents' lack of knowledge about their eligibility for SCHIP.

Another major problem with the program is reflected in the "SCHIP Dip." As illustrated in figure E-4, it is estimated that at least 900,000 children are scheduled to *lose* their SCHIP coverage by 2007 due to reductions in federal funding. Because policymakers knew that it would take the states some time to establish their SCHIP programs and as part of their efforts to balance the federal budget, the $40 billion they initially allocated to fund SCHIP was not distributed equally over the first 10 years. Instead, Congress allocated $4.3 billion per year for the first four years of the program (1998-2001), but then reduced it to $3.15 for the next three years (2002-2004) before having it rise again thereafter. This means that while the number of uninsured children is rising—due to the recession in 2001 and the uneven economic growth the country has experienced thereafter—funding from the federal government is falling. Metaphorically speaking, this resembles the same "Perfect Storm" currently battering Medicaid: growing demand for the program, increasing medical inflation, and declining government revenues.[58]

Figure E-4
The SCHIP Dip: Enrollment and Federal Funding, 1998-2007 (*Projected*)

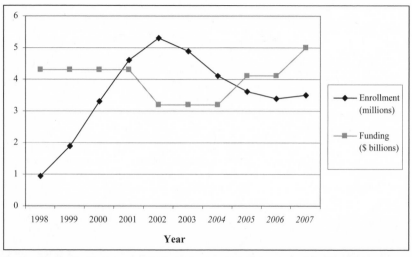

Source: Centers for Medicare and Medicaid Services, U.S. Department of Health and Human Services; Fiscal Year 2003 Analytical Perspectives, White House Office of Management and Budget.

Recognizing this problem, various members of Congress have introduced legislation intended to address the dip and restore funding for SCHIP to the initial levels. But consideration of the bill has been prolonged, which has led to a reduction in federal funding. And as long as the economy sputters along, states will fail to receive sufficient levels of revenue needed to maintain current levels of coverage. This is the weakness of any welfare-style program. Social insurance programs, such as Medicare and Social Security, are virtually impervious to fluctuating economic conditions. They are entitlements on which the government cannot default. SCHIP, however, is a discretionary program. Policymakers can adjust eligibility criteria and benefits in response to larger budgetary pressures (by law states have to balance their budgets annually), even if that means that nearly 1 million children lose their SCHIP coverage over the next three years.

Because of Medicaid and SCHIP's eligibility and financing problems, proponents of universal coverage have traditionally envisioned social insurance (Medicare) to be the optimal vehicle for achieving universal coverage. This enthusiasm for Medicare has persisted despite the fact that the program's managed care experiment in the late 1990s-early 2000s failed, and that it has taken more than a decade of painstaking deliberation and political jockeying just to pass a catastrophic prescription drug plan. But as this book has shown, it's hard to change Medicare. It is a generous, universal, fee-for-service program that—at least from the perspective of its beneficiaries—has been virtually frozen in time from the mid-1960s when there were no "gatekeeping" primary care physicians, prior authorizations, or other restraints from whatever modern medicine had to offer.

Medicare: This *Is* Your (Grand)Father's Health Insurance Program

"I hate this whole G--damn system. I'd blow it up if I could, but I'm stuck with it," said Tom Scully, Administrator for the Centers for Medicare and Medicaid Services (CMS), which operates both programs.

> If it were up to me, I'd buy everybody private insurance and forget about it. Obviously that's what the Republican view is: We ought to do what we do for federal employees—go out and buy every senior citizen a community-rated, structured, and regulated private insurance plan. Let them all go buy an Aetna product, or a Blue Cross product; that's the Republican philosophy. Why should Tom Scully and his staff fix prices for every doctor and hospital in America? Which is what we do.[59]

Prior to 1994, this view of Medicare was practically non-existent outside of a few ideological purists (such as Newt Gingrich) who were rarely in a position of having to govern. The notion that Medicare should be privatized by changing it from a "defined benefit" to a "defined contribution" plan would have been anathema to the leading policymakers in Washington. There was a political consensus about Medicare, as Jonathan Oberlander has documented, that governed the program for the first three decades of its existence. Policymaking was bipartisan in character, even when it involved extraordinary changes to the program's method of reimbursing hospitals and doctors (see chapter 7). Moreover, Republicans and Democrats embraced the idea that Medicare "should be operated as a universal government program, that federal health insurance for the elderly should take the form, in essence, of a single-payer health system."[60]

The 1994 congressional elections, however, triggered a political earthquake: Republicans gained control of both the House of Representatives and the Senate for the first time since 1954. After being out of power for four decades, they had a number of new political agendas, but none bigger than balancing the federal budget. As chapter 7 explains, Medicare was already viewed as a perennial "cash cow" that Congress had been accustomed to using to free up spending for other programs and to achieve some measure of deficit control. But to go beyond deficit control to the next level of actually balancing the budget would have required substantial cuts in Medicare spending that were far beyond the consensus that had existed since the program's beginning.

Conveniently for Republicans, in 1995 Medicare was predicted to begin running a deficit in 2002 and to be completely insolvent by 2032, when the entire "Baby Boom" generation had reached retirement age (see figures E-5, E-6).[61] Republicans responded by proposing $270 billion in Medicare spending reductions over seven years as part of a "Save Medicare" campaign.[62] President Clinton's veto of this and other critical budget legislation passed by the Republicans triggered the famous government shutdown in late 1995-early 1996. President Clinton emerged the political winner from his showdown with House Speaker Newt Gingrich and the House Republicans, and went on to win reelection handily in 1996. In August of 1997, Congress and the President passed the Balanced Budget Act (BBA), which included a number of Medicare reforms and cuts in the program's spending totaling $112 billion over five years.[63]

The centerpiece of the 1997 Medicare reforms was policymakers' creation of Medicare+Choice (M+C), which sought to dramatically increase the number of senior citizens in participating managed care plans.[64] There were already 5 million Medicare beneficiaries enrolled in various managed care plans in 1997 (14 percent of the program's total population), but Republicans had ambitions to significantly increase that number. As Tom Scully previously explained, they wanted to do four things in particular: (1) expand beneficiaries' health care choices; (2) provide additional benefits, such as prescription drug coverage; (3) restrain the growth of federal Medicare spending by encouraging competition among private health plans; and (4) reduce the need for direct government regulation of provider payment policies.[65] In short, Republicans desired to fundamentally change Medicare to a program that provided beneficiaries with a defined contribution towards the purchase of a private health insurance plan.

When M+C was adopted, the Congressional Budget Office predicted that it would eventually enroll 13-15 million individuals or around 34 percent of the entire Medicare population by 2005.[66] Instead, enrollment in M+C peaked at 17% in 1999 (a little more than 6 million beneficiaries) and has since fallen back to less than 12 percent by 2003.[67] Furthermore, of the 346 managed care plans that were participating in M+C in 1998, only 156 were still in the program five years later.[68] The remaining plans have become much less attractive to Medicare beneficiaries, as most have increased premiums and decreased benefits, such as prescription drug coverage.[69]

Ultimately, M+C proved to be an unstable foundation for policymakers to pursue broader reform of the program. Republicans and Democrats disagree over why the M+C initiative failed—either the plans were over-regulated and underpaid by the government or the Medicare population is simply unsuited for profit-oriented managed care.[70] But most would agree that policymakers are left facing a Herculean challenge. They need to find ways to restrain Medicare's costs, while also expanding the program to cover increasingly important but expensive items such as outpatient prescription drugs and nursing home care. And, unfortunately, time is not on their side (figures E-5, E-6).

The risk that a major intergenerational conflict will arise in the future between retirees and workers, who finance retirees' Social Security and Medicare benefits, is considerable. Currently, Medicare takes in increasingly more money by way of the payroll tax than it pays out in benefits, in part because the ratio of workers to retirees is sufficiently high (3.8 to 1) that it generates a surplus of revenue. But this trend will change dramatically beginning in 2011, when the first of the Baby Boomers—the 77 million individuals born between 1946 and 1964—reaches the retirement age of 65. At that point the ratio will have declined to 3.6 workers to each retiree. By 2030, when the last of the Baby Boomers becomes eligible, the ratio will have fallen to 2.3 workers to 1 retiree.[71]

At that point, policymakers will only have three options available to keep Medicare going: increase workers' taxes, decrease beneficiaries' benefits, or some combination of the two. Policymakers could increase the age of eligibility, but it is politically unlikely. This unavoidable future necessity, then, to either increase taxes or decrease Medicare's benefits, made the debate in Congress— over how to *add* an expensive (approximately $500 billion) prescription drug benefit to the program—border on the surreal.[72]

Adding drug coverage to Medicare was fiscally irresponsible, but politically attractive because it benefits the largest and most active voting block in the country: retirees. Coverage of outpatient prescription drugs was not included when Medicare passed in 1965, because it was a relatively insignificant part of medical care at the time. The comparatively few drugs in existence were affordable. But since then prescription drugs have become a critical part of modern medicine's armamentarium. They have also become exceedingly expensive, especially for the elderly, most of whom live on fairly modest fixed incomes.

Consequently, there is nearly unanimous agreement among policymakers that some type of drug benefit needed to be added to Medicare. Yet two-thirds of the program's beneficiaries already had some form of prescription drug coverage (through plans they continued to receive from their previous employers, private Medigap policies, Medicaid, or their enrollment in an M+C plan).[73] So as with all public health insurance initiatives, the trick for policymakers is how to expand the public safety net for those who desperately need help without encouraging employers to curtail their own retiree drug plans and dump the burden on Medicare, thereby driving up the cost to taxpayers and leaving some of the elderly with worse coverage than they have now. While over 60 percent of U.S. companies provided their retirees with health benefits in 1988, less than 35 percent do so today.[74] Policymakers do not want to exacerbate this trend.

This is arguably *the* dilemma facing our nation's health care system, which is half private, half public and has gaps in between: How do policymakers wisely and effectively expand the system's public programs without undercutting the private sector's health insurance arrangements? If the government expands the eligibility of existing public health insurance programs, it could provide too many incentives for businesses to stop providing health coverage as a fringe benefit.

Figure E-5
Medicare's Enrollment (in millions), 1970-2030 (*Projected*)

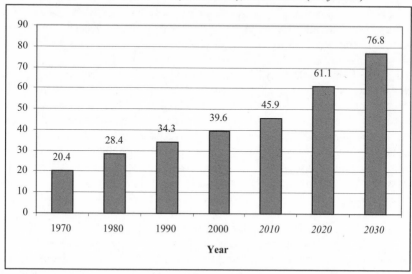

Source: Program Information on Medicare, Medicaid, SCHIP and Other Programs, CMS, 2002.

Figure E-6
Medicare's Trust Fund Balance as % of Annual Costs, 1990-2030 (*Projected*)

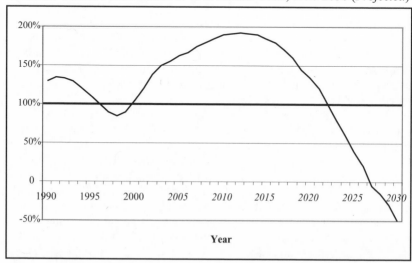

Source: 2003 Trustees' Report; see http://cms.hhs.gov/publications/trusteesreport/2003/figif2.asp

The Medical Malpractice Crisis: Litigation Nation

The previous sections might leave the impression that the only insurance crisis in the U.S. health care system involves the 45 million individuals who don't have coverage. But the nation is currently experiencing another significant insurance problem, which affects physicians and institutional health care providers: professional liability protection (more commonly known as medical malpractice insurance). Its affordability has become an extremely difficult proposition in many parts of the country for physicians in high-risk specialties such as obstetrics, emergency medicine, general surgery, surgical subspecialties (e.g., neurosurgery), and radiology.[75] The crisis has become so bad in some states that thousands of doctors have gone on strike, several hospitals have temporarily closed or threatened to close emergency room, obstetrical or other services, and pregnant women in states such as Washington and Nevada have had to drive as far as seventy miles to find a physician who still delivers babies.[76]

This is actually the country's third medical malpractice crisis. The first, in the early to mid-1970s, was primarily a crisis of insurance availability. As Michelle Mello explains, its distinguishing features were the departure of many major malpractice insurers from the market, which made insurance virtually impossible for many physicians to purchase at any price. This situation led to the formation in many states of insurance companies owned and operated by physicians ("bedpan mutuals") and state-sponsored joint underwriting associations, many of which are still in operation.[77] The second crisis, in the early to mid-1980s, was more a crisis of affordability. Insurers did not pull out of the market, but they began charging premiums that many physicians simply could not afford to pay.[78] Both crises began in much the same way. Physicians in a handful of states experienced a sudden spike in their medical malpractice insurance premiums, which triggered a domino-effect whereby physicians in more and more states found it increasingly difficult to obtain affordable coverage.

The current malpractice insurance crisis is something of a combination of both availability and affordability problems. In 2002, the second largest malpractice carrier in the country, St. Paul Companies, pulled out of the market, partly because of a $940 million underwriting loss in 2001. Several other insurers have subsequently followed its lead. Consequently, many states have witnessed the exiting of insurance companies that held a significant share of the market, which has left thousands of doctors with fewer and much more expensive options for obtaining liability coverage.[79] In some of the hardest hit states such as West Virginia, Pennsylvania, Florida, Nevada and Washington, many physicians have been left without any options whatsoever. No insurance carrier will offer them a policy. Therefore, physicians have had to turn to their states' joint underwriting associations as the "insurer of last resort." Although the purpose of these organizations is to guarantee that all physicians are able to obtain coverage, the rates they charge can and often have been prohibitively high, especially for doctors who have been sued before. In states such as Florida, which do not require that doctors have malpractice insurance, increasing numbers of them are "going bare" and working without coverage. Not surprisingly, "asset protection" is a growing industry in these states, as doctors endeavor to protect their personal property.[80]

The three parties involved—physicians, attorneys, and insurance carriers—all point to each other as the cause of the crisis. Physicians blame "ambulance chasing" attorneys for flooding the courts with frivolous claims that physicians have to either settle prior to going to trial (at the average cost of $30,000) or contest in court (win and still pay on average $95,000). Obviously, both options are money-losers for doctors, even though they win most cases (70 percent are closed without payment).[81] Physicians also blame "out of control" juries who do not understand the realities of medicine, the cumulative effect of multimillion-dollar awards on the cost of health care, and the fact that not all "bad" outcomes are the result of malpractice.[82] The quantity and quality of empirical data on either of these claims is thin. What is clear, though, is that while the number of both claims and awards against doctors has remained relatively steady, the average size of awards has increased substantially.[83]

Insurers concur with physicians in pointing the finger of blame at attorneys. They claim that the large increases in premiums are due to the growing number of "$1 million+" awards, as well as the increases in both the median settlement amount and the average administrative costs associated with defending malpractice claims.[84] Therefore, insurers have joined with physicians in advocating federal legislation, similar to California's law, that limits awards for non-economic damages or "pain and suffering."[85]

Attorneys have responded, perhaps predictably, by blaming both physicians and insurers. They claim that lawsuits are a necessary means of providing victims with the financial support they need to pay for damages inflicted by negligent physicians. When the medical error rate goes down, they argue, so will the rate of litigation.[86] Moreover, attorneys point to insurers' financial practices as the real culprit for skyrocketing premiums. They maintain that insurers underpriced their products in the early 1990s to gain market share against their competitors and in order to invest the premiums they received in the stock market, which annually was producing double-digit returns. But when insurers suffered three straight years of investment losses beginning in 2001, attorneys argue, they had no choice but to substantially increase their premiums to compensate for the effects of a bear market and low bond yields.[87] In other words, attorneys argue, relax. When stocks and bonds recover and new insurers reenter the market to undercut insurance policies that have become too expensive, the "insurance cycle" will repeat itself and today's medical malpractice crisis will disappear just as it did in the 1970s and 1980s.

It is very difficult to empirically test this theory or insurers' and physicians' claims about the causal relationship between lawsuits and premiums. But most observers would agree that our current tort system is not well designed to significantly reduce injuries due to medical errors or to compensate the majority of injured patients in a timely and appropriate way. And because all proposals for tort reform invariably reflect the interests of the three groups that propose them, it is unlikely that meaningful change will occur anytime soon. But what makes the current tort system and its malpractice insurance crisis an impediment to universal coverage is that they both encourage physicians to practice more "defensive medicine," which includes additional and often unnecessary tests to protect them from future lawsuits. Defensive medicine adds billions of dollars to the nation's health expenditures and fuels medical inflation, which only makes health insurance more expensive and increases the number of uninsured.[88]

With so many festering problems in our health care system, perhaps we are approaching another period of serious political deliberation over comprehensive reform. If so, it is critical that policymakers take a moment and learn from previous failures, especially President Clinton's.

Learning from Clinton's Failure: A Decade Later

In the spring of 1993, one year before he died, former President Richard Nixon visited the White House at the invitation of President Clinton. Shortly after he arrived, he pulled Hillary aside and said, "You know, I tried to fix the health care system more than twenty years ago. It has to be done sometime." She replied, "I know, and we'd be better off today if your proposal had succeeded."[89] Ironically, she crafted a plan that closely resembled Nixon's proposal and which ultimately met the same fate: defeat. Reflecting on the outcome ten years later she concluded: "Someday we will fix the system. When we do it, it will be the result of more than fifty years of efforts by Harry Truman, Richard Nixon, Jimmy Carter and Bill and me. Yes, I'm still glad we tried."[90]

Given both the forests of trees and vats of ink consumed analyzing the defeat of health care reform in 1993-94, one pauses before consuming any more (particularly given the attention this book has already paid to it in chapter 7). The only worthwhile purpose this author can see in revisiting Clinton's failure is to relearn some important lessons about the politics of health care reform. Because hope springs eternal and significant problems with our health care system continue to fester, it is likely that there will be another major push for health care reform in the future. Unfortunately, the Clinton effort provides several object lessons in how not to go about it.

Before being criticized, though, the Clintons are to be applauded for having even tried, despite the fact that the likelihood of success was low from the outset. President Clinton was narrowly elected in 1992 in a three-way race in which he ultimately received less than 50 percent of the popular vote. Once in office, his administration had to face an economy in recovery and enormous $200 billion annual budget deficits "as far as the eye could see." Hence, there was little to no room for error and no unused money lying around for major new policy initiatives. Moreover, opting for comprehensive reform—rather than the incremental variety—reduced his administration's chances for success even further.

Nevertheless, the Clintons chose a plan modeled on Republican President Richard Nixon's 1974 health care proposal and built on the same market-oriented strategies that Republicans today desire to impose on Medicare. So there was a chance, however remote, that the Clintons' efforts could have succeeded politically. As Robert Winters, Chairman of Prudential Insurance and Head of the Business Roundtable's Health Care Task Force (which became one of the leading groups opposed to President Clinton's efforts), said: "Were there days when we thought the Clinton plan was going to go through and pass? Oh, yes, absolutely!"[91] At the time, the Democrats controlled the presidency and both houses of Congress. The media was largely sympathetic to the goal of comprehensive reform. Millions of working- and middle-class Americans were without health insurance and millions more lived in fear that they could soon join them. There were many large businesses saddled with enormous health care costs for their workers, and especially their retirees, that desperately wanted major change to the country's health care system. Thus, there was good reason for the abundance of optimism that surrounded the issue of health care reform in 1993.

It is difficult to condense the different explanations for the Clintons' failure into a single coherent argument, but *alienation* is a theme that runs through most of them. In brief, the self-imposed alienation of key policymakers in the Clinton administration (particularly Hillary Clinton and Ira Magaziner) and the extent to which they subsequently alienated key policymakers both in Congress and in the larger health care community led to a health care plan—and a strategy for passing it—that was critically lacking in political feasibility. Hillary Clinton has admitted as much: "After twenty months, we conceded defeat. We knew we had alienated a wide assortment of health care industry experts and professionals, as well as some of our own legislative allies."[92] This alienation, which made passing any kind of reform impossible, unfolded and intensified over time.

The alienation began with the 500+ member President's Task Force on National Health Care Reform that the Clinton administration created in early 1993 for the purposes of drafting a health care proposal. Walter Zelman, a key health policy advisor to the Clintons and a senior member of the Task Force, explains why it was such a mistake: "There are all kinds of ways to make policy. One is to put a small number of people into a back room and have them thrash it out. Another is to have a large, slow, public, participatory effort that builds, you hope, to consensus and public support. We picked the worst of both models, secret and huge. . . . The public—and worse, all kinds of interest groups—saw 500 people behind closed doors, with themselves on the outside."[93] Bob Boorstin, Communications Director for the Task Force, puts it more bluntly:

> What happened with the Health Care Task Force was that it did three things. One, it pissed off the journalists, so they were looking for anything and everything they could find that reflected badly on the process. . . . The second group that it pissed off was the Republican staffers who had burrowed in at HCFA [the Health Care Financing Administration] and OMB [the Office of Management & Budget], particularly at OMB. These people, I mean, the minute they saw an option paper would leak it. So you've got all these headlines in the *Post* and the *Times* and the *Journal* totally based on leaks from Republicans who were holdovers from President Bush and had burrowed into the bureaucracy in order to save their butts, their jobs, their pensions, whatever. So there's a pretty devastating combination. The third group that was really pissed off was the lobbyists. They had no way in. And closing the door in the face of a lobbyist is going to piss them off.[94]

In retrospect, Hillary Clinton agreed that the Task Force was the wrong way to start the policymaking process: "The group was so large that some members concluded they were not at the center of the action where the real work was getting done. Some got frustrated and stopped coming to meetings. Others became narrowly interested in their own piece of the agenda, rather than invested in the outcome of the overall plan. In short, the attempt to include as many people and viewpoints as possible—a good idea in principle—ended up weakening rather than strengthening our position."[95]

The second stage of alienation involved the exclusion of President Clinton's key budget and economic advisors, who would have advocated a less ambitious and more politically feasible proposal for health care reform. Leon Panetta (Director of OMB), Laura D'Andrea Tyson (Chair of the Council of Economic Advisors), Robert Rubin (Chair of the National Economic Council), Lloyd Bentsen (Secretary of the Treasury), and Alice Rivlin (Deputy Director of OMB) had just helped Clinton pass his first budget in August 1993. It proved to be the single biggest and most important accomplishment of the President's first term. The plan required extensive negotiating with numerous members of Congress and difficult political choices, including raising taxes. It passed by one vote in the House and by the tie-breaking vote of Vice President Gore in the Senate. Based on this experience and their professional backgrounds, Clinton's budget and economic advisors were far more knowledgeable than Hillary, Ira Magaziner, or any member of the Health Care Task Force about what was and was not politically feasible. But probably because of the tough questions they would have asked (and later did ask) about the health reform plan, Rivlin claims, they were largely excluded from the Task Force's drafting process.[96] Their lack of input, in Panetta's opinion, damaged the plan's political prospects:

> Instead of the careful work that went into developing the budget, the health care thing became part of a political strategy. . . . The President's plan was designed by a smaller group of individuals. Once it was done, it was very difficult to try to change it. A lot of us indicated our concerns with what would take place. I had kind of a double concern, which was not only the nature of what was being proposed, because it was so hard to understand, but, secondly, I said that the problem is that Congress is not going to be able to understand the implications here. It cannot digest this big a piece of legislation in one bite. I asked, "Who's going to be for this proposal when it goes to Congress?"
>
> In the end, the plan didn't have a lot of useful politics. So the problem is that they lost sight of the fact that without being able to sell it politically, it wasn't going to happen. Unfortunately, of all the battles we'd been through to try to get the budget put in place, all of those lessons just went out the window with the rest of health care reform.[97]

Without the involvement of the administration's key budget and economic advisors, the plan's ambitions were never cross-checked against what realistically could be passed in Congress. The end result, as Robert Rubin points out, was a politically impossible situation: "I think that partly it's because the process led into something that was too large to accomplish at one time. . . . The reform of the health care system in one fell swoop was more than anybody could expect to accomplish."[98]

The last stage of alienation involved key members of Congress and their staff. It was not only senior Republicans, such as Representative Newt Gingrich and Senator Phil Gramm, who were logically and by necessity excluded because of their bitter opposition to any reform whatsoever. Moderate and conservative Democrats, many of whom had extensive backgrounds in health policy, were also ignored. Besides Hillary Clinton and Ira Magaziner's naiveté and hubris, perhaps part of this exclusion can be attributed to the less than helpful advice Hillary claims she received from key senior Democratic members of Congress early in the process:

> We had originally envisioned presenting Congress with an outline of principles that would shape the health care reform legislation. But we subsequently learned that Congressman Dan Rostenkowski expected us to produce a detailed bill, complete with legislative language. Giving Congress a comprehensive bill at the outset turned out to be a tremendous challenge and a tactical mistake for us. We thought it would be 250 pages at most, but as drafting continued, it became clear that the bill needed to be much longer, in part because the plan was complex and in part because we acquiesced to some specific requests from interested groups. . . The Health Security Act delivered by the White House to Congress on October 27 was 1,342 pages long.[99]

But David Abernethy, Staff Director of the House Ways and Means Committee at the time, denies this claim and points to the Clinton administration's lack of Washington experience as a major weakness in moving health care reform along in a timely manner:

> Health care was already receding as a political issue in late '93, in part because the Clinton administration took nine months to get a proposal up to Congress. Mrs. Clinton used to love to say, "Well, your boss, Mr. Rostenkowski, said that we had to send up a bill." The third time she said that to me, I finally said, "Mrs. Clinton, there's a bill and then there's a *bill*. Mr. Rostenkowski did not mean 1,000+ pages of finely dense type. What he meant was that you had to have a reasonably fully fledged-out proposal, so that it was clear what you wanted." I went on to say, "You and I, with all due respect, Mrs. Clinton, could have knocked that out in a weekend."
>
> But they didn't know any better. They were new to Washington. This is a problem with electing a governor and particularly a governor of a small state. A governor of California might be better positioned to understand what it takes to survive in Washington. But they really didn't know. The first meetings with them were painful, just painful.[100]

The Clinton administration and its Democratic allies in Congress did not need—and never would have received—help from most Republican members, but they did need a few, key moderate Republicans for health care reform to be politically feasible. Other than the late Senator John Chafee of Rhode Island, the

Clinton team chose not to seriously engage any Republicans. According to Sheila Burke (Chief of Staff for Republican Senator and Majority Leader Bob Dole), this partisan alienation was a crucial mistake, but also a function of the bitter politics that existed then:

> I think the politics of the time didn't permit it. I think there were a series of decisions that were made that almost precluded . . . our coming to what would have normally been a compromise. I think the decision to exclude the Republicans from the outset was a huge mistake on the part of the White House. . . . Mr. Rostenkowski tried to warn them; Senator Moynihan tried to warn them. But the Democrats had problems on their own side, so that all the pieces that could have been put into place for a compromise had no opportunity. And then it just became too late and too close to the '94 elections. . . .
>
> But at the end of the day you want to solve a problem. There was a history between the House Ways and Means and Senate Finance Committees, where we would often be at opposite ends but there was a commitment—whether it was Dole as Chairman or Packwood, or Bentsen, or Rostenkowski—to come to closure. And we weren't permitted to do that. It was terrible. In the 20 years I've served as a staff member on the Hill, it was by far the worst experience I ever had and I had some horrific experiences. It was *the* worst. It is the period of time I look back on with the greatest regret.[101]

Once the sense of alienation had reached such a high level and affected so many leading representatives of the health care system, comprehensive health reform was effectively dead. Worst of all, making a mid-course correction sometime in 1994—in order for a compromise to be reached over a more modest, incremental reform plan—became politically infeasible as well.

Even millions of middle-class Americans came to feel alienated by the manner in which the Clintons tried to sell their reform plan. "We kept trying to link middle-class concerns to lower-income concerns, knowing that we had an opportunity to piggyback the universal coverage issue onto middle-class insecurities regarding the potential loss of health insurance. But it was a tough sell," argues Zelman. "What the middle class needed was the opportunity to buy health insurance at a reasonable price and then keep it. That could be achieved without universal coverage and without subsidizing insurance for lower-income persons. We kept trying to make a case that anything less than universal coverage would hurt the middle class. But that argument had its limits. It just wasn't true. Every time we made it, we were burning our bridges—there would be no ground left on which to compromise."[102]

Ironically, after the tremendous disappointment over the defeat of health care reform faded over time and the managed care revolution took off with a vengeance in the mid-1990s, some high-ranking Clinton administration officials felt a sense of having been spared politically. They came to believe that if the Clinton health care plan had passed, it would probably have been next to impossible to actually implement and then President Clinton would have been blamed for the hugely unpopular managed care revolution. According to one senior

Clinton administration official, "Implementing the plan would have been a mess. And, so, two things: I think he would have been thrown out [in the '96 election] and his health plan would have been repealed." Laura D'Andrea Tyson, President Clinton's Chair of the Council of Economic Advisors, disagrees with this argument only in that she is skeptical that the plan could even have been implemented before the next presidential election:

> I don't think the health plan would have been implemented by 1996, so I don't agree with the notion that he would have gotten the blame. . . . I think from the time it would have passed in '94 to the time that the '96 election came around not that much could possibly have been done that would have politically affected him. . . . The plan was really complicated. You were going to have to set up all these HIPCs [Health Insurance Purchasing Cooperatives] all over the country. You were going to have to come up with price caps. You were going to have to get the Medicare population enrolled in new plans. When you actually think about doing something that big. . .
>
> What I would say is that if the average American had ever actually been forced to choose among a limited number of health care plans run by regional HIPCs and if their range of medical services had been in any way limited, then, yes, I think it could have been a political disaster because there were some real managed care elements to the Clinton health care plan. But my personal view is that it wouldn't have been feasible to actually implement the plan.[103]

In the end, the failure of health care reform in 1993-94, Abernethy argues, "can be summarized in one sentence: You have to leave the health insurance that most people have alone. You can't come up with a system that requires you to disrupt the existing insurance arrangements that most people have. Even if they aren't very happy with them, they're not going to let you mess with them. The problem with the Clintons' 'managed competition' proposal is that it required the disruption of all existing health insurance arrangements. And that is what the Republicans exploited ruthlessly."[104]

This leaves us with an obvious question: What *can* be done to reach some form of universal coverage and, in the process, improve our current health care system? The final section briefly examines three competing solutions that have recently risen to prominence.

Conclusion: Possible Solutions to the Problem of the Uninsured

Three of the leading proposals for addressing the problem of the uninsured run the gamut from conservative to liberal, modest to ambitious, and Republican to Democratic. The major disagreements between them, Karen Davis and Cathy Schoen explain, are over the role of private insurance in covering the uninsured, whether public programs should be expanded to include additional groups, and the commitment of adequate budgetary resources required to assist those who are unable to afford the full cost of health coverage.[105] Each proposal has its own strengths and weaknesses. Not surprisingly, one proposal's weakness is often another one's strength and vice versa. But to varying degrees they all reflect the limitations highlighted by the Clinton debacle. Structurally, as Abernethy argues, you cannot disrupt the existing health insurance arrangements that most people currently have. And politically, Zelman notes, discretion is the better part of valor: "More than anything else, you have to understand the limitations and restraints—all of them, institutional, political, policy and educational. The opposition will always have more levers, the public can be moved only so much, and you've almost certainly got less power than you think you have."[106]

One option advocated by President George W. Bush calls for tax credits of up to $1,000 for individuals earning below $45,000 a year and $2,000 for families earning below $60,000 a year.[107] Uninsured individuals would use these tax credits to purchase a private health insurance policy. The proposal's primary strength is that it does not call for any new government program or organization, nor does it threaten any existing health insurance arrangements. Therefore, it is the most feasible, modest and least controversial option. However, the proposal has several weaknesses. First, the amount of the tax credits is not enough to purchase an adequate policy, especially given that they would be individual/non-group policies. Since the average cost of a non-group health insurance plan for a family of four is roughly $7,300 per year, even if the tax credit was increased to $3,600, the most generous proposed, the average family would still have to pay about $3,700 out-of-pocket.[108] Given that most of the uninsured are working- to middle-class, this amount would be prohibitively expensive. In addition, the cost of private, individual health insurance policies could increase significantly; employers could use the new policy as an excuse to cease providing health insurance as a fringe benefit; and the credits would have to be paid for by either increased government revenues (more taxes now) or increased government debt (more taxes later).

Another option, advocated by Democratic Representative John Conyers and others, involves significantly expanding Medicare. Citing the high proportion (upwards of 50 percent) of each private health insurance dollar that is diverted to overhead and profits—and, thus, not to cover actual physician and hospital expenses—Marcia Angell, former editor of the *New England Journal of Medicine*, argues that what we need is a national single-payer system that would eliminate unnecessary administrative costs, duplication and profits. In effect, this would be the equivalent of extending Medicare to the entire population. "Medicare is, after all, a government-financed single-payer system embedded within our private, market-based system," notes Angell. "It's by far the most efficient part of our health-care system, with overhead costs of less than 3 percent, and it covers virtually everyone over the age of 65. Medicare is not perfect, but it's the most popular part of the American health-care system."[109] If President Bush's tax-credit proposal is too timid and unlikely to help many uninsured, then the idea of extending Medicare to all suffers from a serious lack of political feasibility. This option was actually considered by Congress in 1994 (see pages 125-127), when the House Ways and Means Committee passed "Medicare Part C." The plan became the leading House alternative to the

Clinton plan. But congressional leaders could not even get it to the floor of the House of Representatives for a vote due to its political impracticality. The extent of the disruption it would cause to existing health insurance institutions and arrangements precludes this option from being seriously considered any time soon. The health care system would have to deteriorate further by several orders of magnitude before a massive expansion of Medicare ("Medicare for All" or "Universal Medicare") would have any chance at passing.

The last, and perhaps most popular, option is something of a middle-ground approach that combines individual obligations and government subsidies. Using the example of automobile insurance, Senator John Breaux (D-LA) and others argue that health insurance should simply be mandatory. According to Senator Breaux, "I'd like to see a nationwide federal mandate that every U.S. citizen purchase a private health insurance policy. There would be a basic plan, that the government would help fund for low-income people who cannot afford it. The government's subsidy would be graduated according to income, to the point where you would ultimately be responsible for paying for it all yourself when you can afford to. People could buy more than the basic plan if they wanted to, but it would be at their expense."[110] One of the keys to this option working is that it would enroll tens of millions of uninsured Americans who are below the age of 35. Mandating that this massive demographic group of young and mostly healthy Americans join the insurance risk pool would drive down the costs for everyone, because they would pay a lot more money into the system in the form of premiums than they would consume in the form of medical care.[111]

Senator Breaux and others ultimately see this option replacing employer-provided insurance over time, which is radical. But as Senator Breaux argues, "Look at the problems we've got in this country right now with employer-sponsored health insurance. Health benefits are among the fastest-growing costs employers face now, and some can't afford to pay for health care any more—many, particularly small businesses, are dropping it entirely. Of course, a lot of people like their employer plan and would want to stay in it. We want to make sure that we don't discourage those who are providing coverage from continuing to do so, if it works for them."[112] According to Ted Halstead, President of the New America Foundation, "The new system would be an improvement for Americans who receive their health insurance from their employers. They would be able to select their own insurance policy and level of coverage from among private providers, instead of being limited to the one selected by their employer. They would also be able to keep the policy and doctors of their choice as they move from job to job. Employers, meanwhile, would not stop paying for coverage—they would simply contribute to the policy of their employee's choosing. After all, employer-subsidized health insurance is voluntary right now, and there is little reason to believe that employers would suddenly stop providing it."[113]

A government mandate for people to purchase their own insurance is an innovative concept, but not a new one. It was part of the Senate Finance Committee's alternative to the Clinton plan in 1994 (see page 127). Similar to the first option of tax credits, an individual mandate does not significantly expand current government programs nor does it create new ones. This feature makes it less threatening to the status quo and, hence, more politically feasible. But an individual mandate has problems of its own. First, it would be enormously expensive. Because two-thirds of the uninsured would need substantial government subsidies to be able to afford an individual health insurance policy, the government would have to provide upwards of $60-$90 billion per year (based on the calculation that 30 million uninsured individuals would need, on average, between $2,000 and $3,000 in government subsidies to help them purchase their insurance policies; in reality, some would need less or none, while others would need a lot more). Moreover, as Jonathan Oberlander points out, an individual mandate plan has no cost-control mechanisms. It relies instead "on the vague hope that competition between private insurers will lower health-care costs. Yet the American experience with competition in medical care provides no basis for relying on a private system—the most expensive in the world, incidentally—to slow health spending. Without government regulation and freed from the negotiating leverage that big companies now exert for premium discounts, there would be no constraints on private insurers who wanted to raise prices. Under an individual mandate program, health-care spending and insurance premiums would continue to escalate, necessitating sizable increases in public subsidies— and likely generating political pressure to retreat from universal coverage."[114]

*   *   *   *

In conclusion, it does not seem likely that universal coverage, the Mount Everest of public policy in the United States, will be conquered any time soon. Maybe individual states, such as Maine and Oregon, will lead the way in innovative policymaking. Maybe it will take a Republican president, willing to risk political martyrdom, to reach across the political aisle and work with Democrats in Congress for comprehensive health care reform to ever pass. Maybe politics will change substantially when the majority of Baby Boomers have retired in the next twenty years and demand the best that modern medicine has to offer. Maybe health care costs, insurance premiums, and the number of uninsured will eventually increase to some critical point (yet to be reached) where sufficient numbers of middle-class voters will finally demand that government do something on their behalf. There is no way to accurately predict, however, what straw will finally break the system's back. But the history of health reform is clear about one thing: despite its numerous shortcomings and failures, which cause immense amounts of suffering for millions of people, our health care system has shown an extraordinary ability to muddle through one crisis after another. In the process, it has successfully repelled every attempt at comprehensive reform. Invariably, then, we are left with the quote from King David that began this epilogue: "But thou, O Lord, how long?"

Notes

1. U.S. Census Bureau, *Income, Poverty and Health Insurance Coverage in the United States: 2003* (Washington: Government Printing Office, August 2004). For full copy of this report, please see: http://www.census.gov/prod/2004pubs/p60-226.pdf (Accessed October 8, 2004).

2. Ibid.

3. Ceci Connolly and Amy Goldstein, "Health Insurance Back as Key Issue," *Washington Post*, March 16, 2003, A05.

4. Robin Toner, "Study Raises Estimate of the Nation's Uninsured," *New York Times*, March 5, 2003.

5. See Robert Pear, "Spending on Health Increased Sharply in 2001," *New York Times*, January 8, 2003; Bradley Strunk, Paul Ginsburg, Jon Gabel, "Tracking Health Care Costs: Growth Accelerates Again in 2001," *Health Affairs* (Web Exclusive: 25 September 2002):W299-W310; US Census Bureau, "Health Insurance Coverage: 2002."

6. Ibid; See also, U.S. Census Bureau, "Health Insurance Coverage: 2002."

7. Stephen Heffler, Sheila Smith, Sean Keehan, M. Kent Clemens, Greg Won, Mark Zezza, "Health Spending Projections for 2002-2012," *Health Affairs* (Web Exclusive: 7 February 2003):W354-W365. See also: Barbara Martinez, "Rate of Increase for Health Costs May Be Slowing," *Wall Street Journal*, June 11, 2003, A1.

8. See "Tracking Health Care Costs," Center for Studying Health System Change (September 2002).

9. See John M. Broder, "Problem of Lost Health Benefits is Reaching Into the Middle Class," *New York Times*, November 25, 2002.

10. Robert Pear, "After Decline, The Number of Uninsured Rose in 2001," *New York Times*, September 30, 2002, A21.

11. White House Office of Management & Budget, *A Citizen's Guide to the Federal Budget, FY 2003* (Washington, D.C.: GPO, February 2002).

12. See Sheryl Gay Stolberg and Robert Pear, "Mysterious Fax Adds to Intrigue Over Drug Bill," *New York Times*, March 18, 2004, A1; John K. Iglehart, "The New Medicare Prescription-Drug Benefit—A Pure Power Play, *New England Journal of Medicine* 350 (February 19, 2004):826-833; John K. Iglehart, "The Dilemma of Medicaid," *New England Journal of Medicine* 348 (May 22, 2003):2140-2148.

13. Elizabeth Warren, Teresa Sullivan, Melissa Jacoby, "Medical Problems and Bankruptcy Problems," Harvard Law School, Public Law Working Paper 8 (April 2000).

14. See U.S. Census Bureau, "Health Insurance Coverage: 2002."

15. Daniel Eisenberg and M. Sieger, "The Doctor is Out," *Time* (June 1, 2003).

16. Michelle Mello, David Studdert, Troyen Brennan, "The New Medical Malpractice Crisis," *New England Journal of Medicine* 348 (June 5, 2003):2281-2284.

17. Ibid.

18. U.S. Census Bureau, *Health Insurance Coverage: 2000* (Washington: U.S. Government Printing Office, September 2001); Robert Pear, "Number of Uninsured Drops for Second Year," *New York Times*, September 28, 2001.

19. See J. Holahan and Mary Beth Pohl, "Changes in Insurance Coverage: 1994-2000 and Beyond," *Health Affairs* (Web Exclusive: 3 April 2002):W162-171.

20. See U.S. Census Bureau, "Health Insurance Coverage: 2002."

21. Leighton Ku, "The Number of Americans Without Health Insurance Rose in 2001 and Appears to be Continuing to Rise in 2002," Center on Budget and Policy Priorities (Washington, D.C.: October 8, 2002).

22. Ibid.

23. David Cho, "Feeling Uninsured About the Future," *Washington Post*, May 16, 2003, B01.

24. Ibid. See also, Jennifer Edwards, Michelle Doty, Cathy Schoen, "The Erosion of Employer-Based Health Coverage and the Threat to Worker's Health Care: Findings from the Commonwealth Fund 2002 Workplace Health Insurance Survey," Commonwealth Fund, August 2002.

25. Pear, "After Decline, the Number of Uninsured Rose in 2001."

26. Alain C. Enthoven, "Employment-Based Health Insurance is Failing: Now What?" *Health Affairs* (Web Exclusive: 28 May 2003):W3237-W3249.

27. James C. Robinson, "The End of Managed Care," *JAMA, Journal of the American Medical Association* 285 (May 23/30, 2001):2622-2628.

28. Joseph B. Treaster, "Aetna Agreement with Doctors Envisions Altered Managed Care," *New York Times*, May 23, 2003.

29. R. Kronick and T. Gilmer, "Explaining the Decline in Health Insurance Coverage, 1979-1995," *Health Affairs* (March/April 1999):30-47.

30. See U.S. Census Bureau, "Health Insurance Coverage: 2001."

31. Chad Terhune, "Fast-Growing Health Plan Has a Catch: $1,000-a-Year Cap," *Wall Street Journal*, May 14, 2003, A1.

32. Ibid.

33. Elizabeth Warren, Teresa Sullivan, Melissa Jacoby, "Medical Problems and Bankruptcy Problems," Harvard Law School, Public Working Paper No. 008 (Norton's Bankruptcy Adviser, May 2000).

34. See Melissa Jacoby, Teresa Sullivan, Elizabeth Warren, "Rethinking the Debates Over Health Care Financing: Evidence from the Bankruptcy Courts," *New York University Law Review* 76 (May 2001):375-412.

35. "A Discussion with Elizabeth Warren," *Harvard Law Today* (March 2002). See http://www.law.harvard.edu/news/today/2002/03/5warren.html (Accessed May 30, 2003).

36. S. Rosenbaum, "Medicaid," *New England Journal of Medicine* 346 (2002):635-640.

37. Iglehart, "The Dilemma of Medicaid," 2140-2148.

38. Diane Rowland and James R. Tallon Jr., "Medicaid: Lessons From a Decade," *Health Affairs* 22 (January/February 2003):138-144.

39. Iglehart, "The Dilemma of Medicaid," 2140-2148.

40. Ibid.

41. Alan Weil, "There's Something About Medicaid," *Health Affairs* 22 (January/February 2003):13-30.

42. Iglehart, "The Dilemma of Medicaid," 2140-2148.

43. Weil, "There's Something About Medicaid," 17. See also B. Bruen and J. Holahan, "Acceleration of Medicaid Spending Reflects Mounting Pressures" (Washington: Kaiser Commission on Medicaid and the Uninsured, May 2002).

44. See Donald J. Boyd, "The Bursting State Fiscal Bubble and State Medicaid Budgets," *Health Affairs* 22 (January/February 2003):46-61; G. Von Behren, N. Samuels, *The Fiscal Survey of States* (Washington, D.C.: National Association of State Budget Officers, November 2002).

45. L. Brown and M. Sparer, "Poor Program's Progress: The Unanticipated Politics of Medicaid Policy," *Health Affairs* 22 (January/February 2003):31-44.

46. Ibid.

47. See Robert Ball's quote in this book on page 81.

48. National Center for Health Statistics, "Table 1.1 Number and Percent of Persons Without Health Insurance Coverage, by Age Group: United States, 1997-2001,"

Early Release of Selected Estimates Based on Data from the 2001 NHIS, July 15, 2002. See http://www.cdc.gov/nchs/about/major/nhis/released200207.htm (Accessed May 6, 2003).

49. Title XIX, Social Security Act.

50. Office of Health Policy, Assistant Secretary for Planning and Evaluation, "Tabulations of the March 1997 Current Population Survey" (Washington: Department of Health and Human Services, December 1997.)

51. James Reschovsky and Peter Cunningham, "CHIPing Away at the Problem of Uninsured Children," *Issue Brief 14* (Washington, D.C.: Center for Studying Health System Change, August 1998).

52. Centers for Medicare and Medicaid Services, "State Child Health Insurance Program Plan Activity Map," updated as of August 6, 2002. For more information, see http://www.cms.hhs.gov/schip/chip-map.asp (Accessed September 26, 2002).

53. See Marsha Gold, Jessica Mitler, Debra Draper, David Rousseau, "Participation of Plans and Providers in Medicaid and SCHIP Managed Care," *Health Affairs* 22 (January/February):230-240.

54. Jennifer M. Ryan, "SCHIP Turns Five: Taking Stock, Moving Ahead," National Health Policy Forum, Issue Brief No. 781 (George Washington University: August 15, 2002).

55. Embry Howell, Ruth Almeida, Lisa Dubay, Genevieve Kenney, "Early Experience with Covering Uninsured Parents Under SCHIP," Series A, No. A-51, Urban Institute (Washington, D.C.: May 2002).

56. Ian Hill, Amy Westpfahl Lutzky, "Is There a Hole in the Bucket? Understanding SCHIP Retention," Assessing the New Federalism, Occasional Paper No. 67 (Urban Institute: May 2003).

57. Ibid.

58. See Weil, "There's Something About Medicaid," 18-19.

59. Tom Scully interview with the author, October 24, 2002.

60. See Jonathan Oberlander, *The Political Life of Medicare* (Chicago: The University of Chicago Press, 2003), Chapter 7, 157-196. Oberlander's book is the best analysis of the history and politics of Medicare.

61. Ibid., 172-173.

62. George Hager, "Medicare is Targeted for Large Cuts," *Congressional Quarterly*, April 8, 1995, 1013.

63. Charles N. Kahn and Hanns Kuttner, "Budget Bills and Medicare Policy: The Politics of the BBA," *Health Affairs* 18 (January/February 1999):37-47.

64. Brian Biles, Geraldine Dallek, Andrew Dennington, "Medicare+Choice After Five Years: Lessons for Medicare's Future: Findings From Seven Major Cities," The Commonwealth Fund and the George Washington University Medical Center, Field Report (September 2002).

65. Ibid., 1.

66. S. Christensen, "Medicare+Choice Provisions in the Balanced Budget Act of 1997," *Health Affairs* (July/August 1998):225-231.

67. Marsha Gold, "Can Managed Care and Competition Control Medicare Costs," *Health Affairs* (Web Exclusive: 2 April 2003):W3-177.

68. Ibid.

69. L. Achman, M. Gold, *Trends in Medicare+Choice Benefits and Premiums, 1999-2002* (New York: Commonwealth Fund, 2002).

70. M. Angell, "Dr. Frist to the Rescue," *American Prospect* 14 (February 1, 2003).

71. Paul J. Feldstein, *Health Policy Issues: An Economic Perspective on Health Reform* (Chicago: AUPHA Press, 1999), 84-85.

72. Robin Toner, Robert Pear, "House Committees Set Off Bitter Battle Over Medicare," *New York Times*, June 18, 2003, A20.

73. Oberlander, *The Political Life of Medicare*, 192.

74. See Editorial, "The Medicare Momentum," *New York Times*, June 16, 2003, A22; "A Corporate Push to Cut the Cost of Retirees' Drugs," *New York Times*, July 2, 2003, A1.

75. Mello, Studdert, Brennan, "The New Medical Malpractice Crisis," 2281. This section borrows heavily from Mello, Studdert, and Brennan's excellent article.

76. Ibid. See also, Sarah Kershaw, "In Insurance Cost, Woes for Doctor and Women," *New York Times*, May 29, 2003.

77. Mello, Studdert, Brennan, "The New Medical Malpractice Crisis," 2281. See also, Rick Mortimer, "What's Happening to the Cost and Quality of Medical Malpractice Insurance," *Cost and Quality Journal* (March 1998).

78. See Stephen Zuckerman, "Medical Malpractice: Claims, Legal Costs, and The Practice of Defensive Medicine," *Health Affairs* 3 (1988):128-134.

79. Mello, Studdert, Brennan, "The New Medical Malpractice Crisis," 2282.

80. Ibid.

81. See Feldstein, *Health Policy Issues*, Chapter 13, 137-148; Jennifer Barrett, "How to Fix the Medical Liability System," *Newsweek Web Exclusive* (February 6, 2003) See http://stacks.msnbc.com/news/869706.asp?cp1=1 (Accessed June 3, 2003).

82. Mello, Studdert, Brennan, "The New Medical Malpractice Crisis," 2283.

83. U.S. Department of Health and Human Services, "Confronting the New Health Care Crisis: Improving Health Care Quality and Lowering Costs by Fixing our Medical Liability System," (Washington, D.C.: Government Printing Office, July 25, 2002). See http://aspe.hhs.gov/daltcp/reports/litrefm.htm (Accessed June 20, 2003).

84. Lawrence E. Smarr, "Statement of the Physician Insurers Association of America," United States Senate Judiciary Committee and Health, Education, Labor and Pensions Committees, February 11, 2003. See http://www.thepiaa.org/pdf_files/February_11_Testimony.pdf (Accessed June 20, 2003).

85. See Jyoti Thottam, "A Chastened Insurer," *Time* (June 1, 2003); Barrett, "How to Fix the Medical Liability System."

86. Mello, Studdert, Brennan, "The New Medical Malpractice Crisis," 2283.

87. See M. Crane, "A New 'Malpractice Crisis'? Malpractice Rates are Soaring Again," *Medical Economics* 9 (2001):133; P. Greve, "Anticipating and Controlling Rising Malpractice Insurance Costs," *Healthcare Financial Management* 56 (2002):50-56.

88. Feldstein, *Health Policy Issues*, 140.

89. Hillary Clinton, *Living History* (New York: Simon & Schuster, 2003), 226.

90. Ibid., 249.

91. Robert Winters interview with the author, August 28, 2002.

92. Clinton, *Living History*, 247.

93. Walter Zelman and Lawrence D. Brown, "Interview: Looking Back on Health Care Reform: 'No Easy Choices'," *Health Affairs* 17 (November/December 1998):61-68.

94. Bob Boorstin interview with the author, January 5, 2003.

95. Clinton, *Living History*, 153.

96. Alice Rivlin interview with the author, August 12, 2002.

97. Leon Panetta interview with the author, August 13, 2002.

98. Robert Rubin interview with the author, November 12, 2002.

99. Clinton, *Living History*, 191.

100. David Abernethy interview with the author, June 19, 2002.

101. Sheila Burke interview with the author, October 2, 2002.

102. Zelman and Brown, "Interview: Looking Back on Health Care Reform: 'No Easy Choices'," 63.

103. Laura D'Andrea Tyson interview with the author, September 30, 2002.

104. Abernethy interview with the author.

105. Karen Davis and Cathy Schoen, "Creating Consensus on Coverage Choices," *Health Affairs* (Web Exclusive: 23 April 2003):W3199.

106. Zelman and Brown, "Interview: Looking Back on Health Care Reform: 'No Easy Choices'," 67.

107. U.S. Department of the Treasury, *General Explanations of the Administration's Fiscal Year 2004 Revenue Proposals* (Washington: Treasury Department, February 2003).

108. Marcia Angell, "Insufficient Credits," *The American Prospect* 12 (September 2001).

109. Marcia Angell, "The Forgotten Domestic Crisis," *New York Times*, October 13, 2002.

110. Gail R. Wilensky, "Interview: Thinking Outside the Box: A Conversation with John Breaux," *Health Affairs* (Web Exclusive: 5 March 2003):W3124-W3130.

111. Ted Halstead, "To Guarantee Universal Coverage, Require It," *New York Times*, January 31, 2003.

112. Wilensky, "Interview: Thinking Outside the Box: A Conversation with John Breaux," W3125.

113. Halstead, "To Guarantee Universal Coverage, Require It."

114. Jonathan Oberlander, "One Dimensional," *The American Prospect* (Web Feature: February 2003).

BIBLIOGRAPHY

Congressional Hearings and Reports

"1989 Report of the Physician Payment Review Commission (PPRC)," *Hearings before the Subcommittee on Health of the Committee on Ways and Means*, House of Representatives, 101st Congress, 1st Session (March 21, 1989).

Conference on the Future of Medicare, Committee on Ways and Means, U.S. House of Representatives, 98th Congress, 1st Session (November 29, 1983).

"Future Directions in Social Security," *Hearings before the Senate Special Committee on Aging*, 93rd Congress, 1st Session (Washington, D.C.: GPO, 1973).

"Health Care Cost Containment Strategies," *Hearings Before the Committee on Labor and Human Resources*, U.S. Senate, 98th Congress, 2nd Session (June 21, 1984).

"Hospital Prospective Payment System," *Hearings before the Subcommittee of the Committee on Finance*, U.S. Senate, 98th Congress, 1st Session (February 17, 1983).

"Medicare: A Fifteen-Year Perspective," *Hearings before the Select Committee on Aging*, House of Representatives, 96th Congress, 2nd Session (July 30, 1980), comm. Pub. No. 96-258.

Medicare and Health Care Chartbook, Committee on Ways and Means, U.S. House of Representatives, 105th Congress, 1st Session (Washington, D.C.: GPO, 1997).

"Medicare and Medicaid Budget Priorities in the 1990s," *Hearings before the Select Committee on Aging*, House of Representatives, 101st Congress, 1st Session (March 23, 1989).

"Medicare and Medicaid," *Hearings before the Subcommittee on Health of the Committee on Finance*, U.S. Senate, 100th Congress, 1st Session (January 29, 1987).

"Medicare and Medicaid: Problems, Issues, and Alternatives," Report of the Staff to the Committee on Finance, U.S. Senate (Washington, D.C.: GPO, 1970).

"Medicare at the Crossroads," *Hearing before the Subcommittee on Health and Long-Term Care of the Select Committee on Aging*, House of Representatives, 98th Congress 1st Session (June 1983).

"Medicare Hospital Prospective Payment System," *Hearings before the Subcommittee on Health of the House Committee on Ways and Means*, 98th Congress, 1st Session (February 14-15, 1983).

"Medicare's Prospective Payment System: Strategies for Evaluating Cost, Quality, and Medical Technology," Office of Technology Assessment, U.S. Congress (Washington, D.C.: GPO, 1985).

"National Health Insurance Proposals," *Hearings before the Committee on Ways and Means*, House of Representatives, 92nd Congress, 1st Session (October 19-20, 1971), 287-89.

"National Health Insurance," *Hearings before the Committee on Ways and Means*, House of Representatives, 93rd Congress, 2nd Session, vol. 2 (April 24, 25, and 26, 1974).

"National Health Insurance," *Hearings before the Committee on Ways and Means*, House of Representatives, 93rd Congress, 2nd Session, vol. 3 (May 3, 10, and 17, 1974).

"Payroll Taxes, Health Insurance, and SBA Budget Proposals," *Hearings before the Committee on Small Business*, House of Representatives, 101st Congress, 2nd Session (March 29, 1990).

"Prospects for Medicare's Hospital Insurance Trust Fund," prepared by the Congressional Budget Office for the Special Committee on Aging, U.S. Senate, 98th Congress, 1st Session (Washington, D.C.: GPO, 1983).

"Social Security Act Amendments of 1949," *Hearings before the House Committee on Ways and Means* (Washington, D.C.: GPO, 1949), part 2.

"Status of the Medicare Hospital Prospective Payment System," *Hearing before the Subcommittee on Health of the Committee on Ways and Means*, U.S. House of Representatives, 100th Congress, 2nd Session (March 1, 1988).

Government, Private, and Miscellaneous Documents and Publications

1973 Annual Report of the Board of Trustees of the Federal Old-Age Insurance and Survivors Insurance and Disability Insurance Trust Funds (Washington, D.C.: GPO, 1974).

1976 Annual Report of the Board of Trustees of the Federal Old-Age Insurance and Survivors Insurance and Disability Insurance Trust Funds (Washington, D.C.: GPO, 1977).

"1990 National Executive Poll on Health Costs & Benefits," *Business & Health* (April 1990).

AARP, Interoffice Memorandum (August 12, 1994).

———. Press Release, "It's Time for Health Care Reform" (August 11, 1994).

"Address before a Joint Session of the Congress on the State of the Union, January 25, 1994," *Weekly Compilation of Presidential Documents*, vol. 30 (January 31, 1994).

Board of Trustees, Federal Hospital Insurance Trust Fund, *1983 Annual Report on Federal Hospital Insurance Trust Fund*, House Committee on Ways and Means, 98th Congress, 1st Session (Washington, D.C.: GPO, 1983).

Budget of the United States Government, Executive Office of the President, Fiscal Year 1981.

"The Case for National Health Insurance," *AFL-CIO American Federationist* (January 1970).

"The Committee on the Costs of Medical Care," *Journal of the American Medical Association* 99 (December 3, 1932).

Centers for Medicare and Medicaid Services, "State Child Health Insurance Program Plan Activity Map."

Committee on Ways and Means, *Health Care Reform: Chairman's Mark* (June 10, 1994).

Congressional Budget Office, *Analysis of the Administration's Health Proposal* (Washington, D.C.: GPO, February 1994).

————. *A Preliminary Analysis of Senator Mitchell's Health Proposal* (Washington, D.C.: GPO, August 9, 1994).

————. *Profile of Health Care Coverage* (Washington, D.C.: GPO, March 1979).

Eisenhower to E. F. Hutton (October 7, 1953), Central Files Box 848, File 156-C; Dwight D. Eisenhower Presidential Library, Abilene, Kans.

Employee Benefit Research Institute, *Sources of Health Insurance and Characteristics of the Uninsured: Analysis of the March 1992 Current Population Survey* (Washington, D.C.: EBRI, 1993).

————. *Sources of Health Insurance and Characteristics of the Uninsured* (Washington, D.C.: EBRI, January 1994).

"Expenditures for Health Care: Federal Programs and Their Effects," Congressional Budget Office (Washington, D.C.: GPO, 1977).

"Factors that Impede Progress in Implementing the Health Maintenance Organization Act of 1973" (Washington, D.C.: GAO, September 3, 1976).

"Fetter, Thompson: Inventors of DRG's Look at PPS Now," *Hospitals* (July 5, 1992).

The Fourth Annual A. Foster Higgins Health Care Benefits Survey (New York: A. Foster Higgins, 1989).

Gibbons, Sam M., "The Chairman's Health Care Reform Mark, Summary," Committee on Ways and Means (June 6, 1994).

Group Health Association of America, *Patterns in HMO Enrollment* (Washington, D.C.: 1992).

Health Insurance Association of America, and KPMG Peat Marwick Survey, *Washington Post*, June 16, 1998, C3.

————. *Source Book of Health Insurance Data* (Washington, D.C.: Health Insurance Association of American, 1991).

"Health Insurance: Cost Increases Lead to Coverage Limitations and Cost Shifting," (Washington, D.C.: General Accounting Office, May 1990).

The Henry J. Kaiser Family Foundation, "Health Reform Legislation: A Comparison of House & Senate Majority Leadership Bills" (August 1994).

"History of the Rising Costs of the Medicare and Medicaid Programs and Attempts to Control These Costs: 1966-1975," Department of Health, Education, and Welfare (Washington, D.C.: General Accounting Office, 1976).

"House Democratic Healthcare Reform Bill as of August 10, 1994," Federal Health Update (August 10, 1994).

Inland Steel Company v. United Steel Workers of America (CIO), 77 NLRB 4 (1948).

Inland Co. v. NLRB, U.S. Court of Appeals, 7th Circuit (September 23, 1948).

Interdepartmental Committee to Coordinate Health and Welfare Activities, *The Nation's Health* (Washington, D.C.: GPO, 1939).

Journal of the American Medical Association 78 (1922).

Lewin-VHI, "Expanding Insurance Coverage without a Mandate" (Lewin-VHI: May 18, 1994).

Mercer/Foster Higgins; U.S. Bureau of Labor Statistics, *Nation's Business* (July 1998).

"National Health Insurance: Diagnosing the Alternatives," *AFL-CIO American Federationist* (June 1974), 7.

"National Health Security: A Clear Answer," *AFL-CIO American Federationist* (June 1971).

National Health Insurance (Washington, D.C.: AEI Press, November 13, 1974).

Office of Health Policy, Assistant Secretary for Planning and Evaluation, "Tabulations of the March 1997 Current Population Survey" (Washington: Department of Health and Human Services, December 1997).

Organization for Economic Cooperation and Development, *Health Care Reform: The Will to Change* (Paris: OECD, 1996).

———. *Health Care Systems in Transition* (Paris: OECD, 1990).

———. *The Reform of Health Care Systems* (Paris: OECD, 1994).

———. *Social Expenditure 1960-90* (Paris: OECD, 1985).

"Physician Payment Reform: Prospects for the Future," *Business & Health* (July 1987).

Prospective Payment Assessment Commission (ProPAC), *Medicare and the American Health Care System: Report to the Congress* (Washington, D.C.: 1985-1997).

Public Papers of the President: Lyndon B. Johnson, 1965 (Washington, D.C.: GPO, 1966).

"The Rapid Rise of Hospital Costs," Executive Office of the President's Council on Wage and Price Stability Staff Report (Washington, D.C.: GPO, January 1977).

"Recollections (Discussions) by Social Security Administration Officials' Knowledge and/or Involvement in Certain Stages of Early Implementation of the Medicare Program (Calendar Year 1966), SSA Regional Office, Atlanta (September 25, 1992), provided to the author by Mr. Arthur Hess.

Report of the 1979 Advisory Council on Social Security, U.S. House of Representatives (Washington, D.C.: GPO, 1980).

Report of the 1982 Advisory Council on Social Security (Washington, D.C.: GPO, 1983).

"Report of the Physician Payment Review Commission; and Fiscal Year 1988 Budget Issues Related to Physician Payment under the Medicare Program," *Hearing Before the Subcommittee on Health of the Committee on Ways and Means*, House of Representatives, 100th Congress, 1st Session (March 3, 1987).

"The Right to Health Care," *AFL-CIO American Federationist* (September 1972).

S. 545, 81st Congress, 1st Session.

S. 1581, S. 1456, 81st Congress, 1st Session.

S. 1620, 76th Congress, 1st Session.

S. 1970, H.R. 4924, 81st Congress, 1st Session.

Smarr, Lawrence E., "Statement of the Physician Insurers Association of America," United States Senate Judiciary Committee and Health, Education, Labor and Pensions Committee, February 11, 2003.

"Social Security Amendments of 1983," P.L. 98-21.

"Summary: Senate Committee on Labor and Human Resources Health Care Reform Mark as of June 9, 1994," from the Office of Senator Edward M. Kennedy.

"Statement by the AFL-CIO Executive Council on National Health Insurance," Bal Harbour, Florida (February 20, 1967).

U.S. Bureau of the Census, *Current Population Reports: 1979*, Series P-60, No. 130, 3.

———. "Statistical Abstract of the United States" (Washington, D.C.: GPO, 1992).

U.S. Census Bureau, *Health Insurance Coverage: 2000* (Washington: Government Printing Office, September 2001).

U.S. Census Bureau, *Health Insurance Coverage: 2001* (Washington: Government Printing Office, September 2002).

U.S. Department of Health, Education, and Welfare, *Facts about the Hill-Burton Program, July 1, 1947-June 30, 1971* (Washington, D.C.: GPO, 1972).

U.S. Department of Health and Human Services, "Confronting the New Health Care Crisis: Improving Health Care Quality and Lowering Costs by Fixing our Medical Liability System," (Washington, D.C.: Government Printing Office, July 25, 2002).

U.S. Department of the Treasury, *General Explanations of the Administration's Fiscal Year 2004 Revenue Proposals* (Washington: Treasury Department, February 2003).

U.S. Interdepartmental Committee to Coordinate Health and Welfare Activities, *Proceedings of the National Health Conference* (Washington, D.C.: GPO, 1939).

Vital Speeches of the Day, vol. 3 (New York: The City News Pub. Co., October 15, 1936).

White House Office of Management & Budget, *A Citizen's Guide to the Federal Budget, FY 2003* (Washington, D.C.: Government Printing Office, February 2002).

Oral History Interviews

Edward Berkowitz, HCFA Oral History Interviews (1995-96): http://www.ssa.gov/history/ Joseph Califano, Hale Champion, Jay Constantine, Bob Derzon, William Fullerton, and William Hsiao.

David Abernethy, personal interview with the author, June 19, 2002.

Interview with Arthur Altmeyer, Oral History Collection, Columbia University (1965).

Bob Boorstin, personal interview with the author, January 5, 2003.

Interview with James Brindle and Martin Cohen, Oral History Collection, Columbia University (1967).

Sheila Burke, personal interview with the author, October 2, 2002.

Interview with Blue Carstenson, Oral History Collection, Columbia University (1966).

Representative Jim Cooper, personal interview with the author, August 23, 2002.

Interview with Nelson Cruikshank, Oral History Collection, Columbia University (1966).

Nancy-Ann DeParle, personal interview with the author, November 4, 2002.

Interview with Martha Eliot, Oral History Collection, Columbia University (1965).

Interview with Katherine Ellickson, Oral History Collection, Columbia University (1969).

Alain Enthoven, personal interview with the author, August 14, 2002.

Jack Faris, personal interview with the author, August 15, 2002.

Judith Feder, personal interview with the author, July 31, 2002.

Interview with Aime Forand, Oral History Collection, Columbia University (1965).

Sherry Glied, personal interview with the author, November 30, 2002.

Interview with Arthur Hess, Oral History Collection, Columbia University (1968).

Interview with Leonard Lesser, Oral History Collection, Columbia University (1966).

Interview with Leonard Lesser and Lisbeth Bamberger Schorr, Oral History Collection, Columbia University (1969).

Mills, Wilbur, Oral History Interviews (November 2, 1971 and March 25, 1987), by Joe B. Frantz and Michael L. Gillette, respectively, Lyndon B. Johnson Presidential Library.

Interview with Robert Myers, Oral History Collection, Columbia University (1967).

Interview with Robert R. Neal, Oral History Collection, Columbia University (1967).

John Ong, personal interview with the author, August 23, 2002.

Leon Panetta, personal interview with the author, August 13, 2002.

Interview with Claude Pepper, Oral History Collection, Columbia University (1968).

Interview with Allen Pond, Oral History Collection, Columbia University (1966).

Lisa Potetz, personal interview with the author, July 24, 2002.

Robert Reischauer, personal interview with the author, August 16, 2002.

Interview with Elliot Richardson, Oral History Collection, Columbia University (1967).

Alice Rivlin, personal interview with the author, August 12, 2002.

Dan Rostenkowski, personal interview with the author, June 25, 2002.

Robert Rubin, personal interview with the author, November 12, 2002.

Tom Scully, personal interview with the author, October 24, 2002.

Representative Pete Stark, personal interview with the author, June 5, 2002.
Laura D'Andrea Tyson, personal interview with the author, September 30, 2002.
Bruce Vladeck, personal interview with the author, August 14, 2002.
Representative Henry Waxman, personal interview with the author, September 3, 2002.
Interview with Elizabeth Wickenden, Oral History Collection, Columbia University (1967).
Gail Wilensky, personal interview with the author, August 7, 2002.
Interview with Alanson Willcox, Oral History Collection, Columbia University (1965).
Caspar Weinberger, personal interview with the author, September 5, 1998.
Robert Winters, personal interview with the author, August 28, 2002.

Newspaper, Magazine, and Congressional Quarterly Articles

"A Long Look at the SSS." *Wall Street Journal*, July 15, 1974, editorial, 10.
"Aetna Agreement with Doctors Envision Altered Managed Care," *New York Times*, May 23, 2003.
"After Decline, the Number of Uninsured Rose in 2001," *New York Times*, September 30, 2002, A21.
"Agreed: Here Comes National Health Insurance," *New York Times Magazine*, July 21, 1974, 10.
"AMA Chief Fishbein Praises Hospital Program." *New York Times*, December 31, 1939, 21.
"AMA Open to Compromise on a Plan for Health Insurance." *New York Times*, October 8, 1974.
"Brief Descriptions of 7 Major Health Insurance Programs Considered in 1974." *1974 CQ Almanac* (Washington, D.C.: GPO), 388-89.
"CBO Turns Budget Spotlight on Health-Care Overhaul." *Congressional Quarterly Weekly Report* 52 (February 12, 1994), 290-91.
"Clinton Move on Health Divides Hill Coalitions." *Washington Post*, August 5, 1994, A1.
"Congress Lags on Health Insurance." *New York Times*, May 27, 1974, 52.
Congressional Quarterly, *Presidency 1975* (Washington, D.C.: CQ Press, March 1976).
"The Doctor is Out," *Time*, June 1, 2003.
"Doubt Surfaces on Bill Passage as Senate Struggle Continues." *Congressional Quarterly Weekly Report* 52 (August 20, 1994), 2458.
"Drive for Health Bill This Session Intensifies." *Washington Post*, August 14, 1974, A8.
"Endless Ramifications," *Washington Post*, August 1, 1994, A25.
"Fast-Growing Health Plan Has a Catch: $1,000-a-Year Cap," *Wall Street Journal*, May 14, 2003, A1.
"Feeling Uninsured About the Future," *Washington Post*, May 16, 2003, B01.
"For Health Care, Time Was a Killer." *New York Times*, August 29, 1994, A1.
"Ford Rating in Poll Slips to Low of 42%." *New York Times*, December 26, 1974, 1.
"The Forgotten Domestic Crisis," *New York Times*, October 13, 2002.
"Gibbons' Patched-Together Health Bill Now Faces Test on the Floor." *Congressional Quarterly Weekly Report* 52 (July 2, 1994), 1793.
"A Health Bill That Wasn't and Why." *Medical World News*, September 13, 1974, 17.
"Health Bill: One More Try." *Washington Post*, August 6, 1974, A11.
"Health Bill Seen Dead This Year." *Washington Post*, August 22, 1974, A1.
"Health Care Cost Growth Slowing Down: Trend May Dampen Prospects for Reform." *Washington Post*, December 22, 1993, A1.

"The Health Care Debate." *New York Times*, July 20, 1994, A1.

"Health Care Reform: The Collapse of a Quest." *Washington Post*, October 11, 1994, A6.

"Health Care Now: On a Cold Day in 1971." President Richard M. Nixon's Speech to Congress, February 18, 1971; excerpts, *The New Republic*, September 19, 1994, 11.

"The Health Hearings." *New York Times*, June 11, 1939, part 4, editorial, 8.

"The Health Insurance Debate." *Washington Post*, May 26, 1974, editorial, C6.

"Health Insurance Back as a Key Issue," *Washington Post*, March 16, 2003, A05.

"Health Insurance Favored By Millions." *New York Times*, January 22, 1939, 9.

"Health Insurance: Hearings on New Proposals." *Congressional Quarterly Almanac* (Washington, D.C.: CQ Press, 1971), 541-54.

"Health Insurance: No Action in 1974." *Congressional Quarterly Almanac* (Washington, D.C.: CQ Press, 1974), 386-94.

"Health Insurance Package Unveiled by Wilbur Mills." *Washington Post*, August 15, 1974, 1.

"Health Plan Will Swell Deficit, Hill Office Says." *Washington Post*, February 9, 1994, A1.

"Hospital Consolidation." *New York Times*, April 30, 1989, 24.

"House Approves Plan to Shore Up Social Security." *Washington Post*, March 10, 1983, A1.

"House Committees Set Off Bitter Battle Over Medicare," *New York Times*, June 18, 2003, A20.

"House Letting Senate Go First." *New York Times*, August 5, 1994, A1.

"In Insurance Cost, Woes for Doctor and Women," *New York Times*, May 29, 2003.

"Insuring the National Health." *Newsweek* , June 3, 1974, 73.

"Kennedy Losing Some Support on Health Aid Bill." *Washington Post*, April 17, 1974, A20.

"Key Committees Bear Down on Overhaul Proposals." *CQ Weekly Report*, June 11, 1994, 1521-22.

"Labor Flexes Its Legislative Muscle." *Nation's Business*, January 1975, 58.

"Labor Hardens Opposition to Compromise Health Bill." *Washington Post*, April 30, 1974, A2.

"Labor Turns Up Heat on Senate Health-Care Bill." *Wall Street Journal*, August 5, 1994, 3.

"Letters to the Editor: Labor's Case for Health Legislation." *Washington Post*, July 5, 1974, A17.

"Medical Costs Are Increasing at a Low Rate: Studies Show Slowest Pace in 20 Years." *Wall Street Journal*, July 14, 1994, 2.

"Medicare is Targeted for Large Cuts," *Congressional Quarterly*, April 8, 1995.

"The Medicare Momentum," *New York Times*, Editorial, June 16, 2003, A22.

"Mills Panel Drafts New Plan." *Washington Post*, August 20, 1974, A1.

"National Health Program Offered By Wagner." *New York Times*, March 1, 1939, 1.

"National Health Bill." *New York Times*, March 12, 1939, Part IV.

"National Health Insurance." *1975 Congressional Quarterly Almanac* (Washington, D.C.: GPO, 1976), 636.

"National Health Insurance: Here Comes the Main Event." *Medical World News*, March 1, 1974, 15.

"National Health Insurance Is on the Way." *Business Week*, January 26, 1974, 70.

"Nixon's Health Insurance Plan Going to the Hill." *Washington Post*, January 9, 1974, A1.

"Nixon Presses Health Plan: Would Accept Compromise." *Washington Post*, May 21, 1974, A4.
"Nixon Sees Passage in '74 of Health Insurance Plan." *New York Times*, February 6, 1974, 16.
"No Kidding, Mr. Meany." *Wall Street Journal*, August 23, 1974, editorial, 6.
"Number of Uninsured Drops for Second Year," *New York Times*, September 28, 2001.
"Problem of Lost Health Benefits is Reaching Into the Middle Class," *New York Times*, November 25, 2002.
"Rethinking the Goals of Clinton Reform." *Business Insurance*, October 25, 1993, 2.
"Roosevelt Plans to Build Hospitals for Needy Regions." *New York Times*, December 23, 1939.
"Senate Votes Aged Aid Rescue Bill." *Washington Post*, March 24, 1983, A1.
"Social Security: Promising Too Much to Too Many?" *U.S. News & World Report*, July 15, 1974, 26-30.
"Spending on Health Increased Sharply in 2001," *New York Times*, January 8, 2003.
"Study Raises Estimate of the Nation's Uninsured," *New York Times*, March 5, 2003.
"To Guarantee Universal Coverage, Require It," *New York Times*, January 31, 2003.
"Wagner's Health Bill Result of Long Drive." *New York Times*, March 5, 1939, Part 4.
"Walkout on Health." *New York Times*, August 23, 1974, editorial, 28.
"Ways and Means Panel with Mills Gone." *Wall Street Journal*, December 11, 1974, 4.
"Weakened Mills and His Committee Face Rough Going." *Wall Street Journal*, November 29, 1974, 1.
"White House Attacks Critics on Health Care." *Wall Street Journal*, July 25, 1994, 2.

Books and Journal Articles

Aaron, Henry S., ed. *The Problem That Won't Go Away: Reforming U.S. Health Care Financing*. Washington, D.C.: The Brookings Institution, 1996.
Achenbaum, Andrew. *Social Security: Visions and Revisions*. Cambridge: Cambridge University Press, 1986.
Achman, L., M. Gold. *Trends in Medicare+Choice Benefits and Premiums, 1999-2002*. New York: Commonwealth Fund, 2002.
Alford, Robert. *Health Care Politics: Ideological and Interest Group Barriers to Reform*, Chicago: University of Chicago Press, 1975.
Altman, Drew. "The Realities Behind the Polls," *Health Affairs* 14 (Spring 1995): 24-26.
Altmeyer, Arthur. *The Formative Years of Social Security*. Madison: University of Wisconsin Press, 1968.
Anderson, Odin. *Blue Cross since 1929*. Cambridge: Ballinger Publishing Co., 1975.
———. *The Uneasy Equilibrium: Private and Public Financing of Health Services in the United States, 1875-1965*. New Haven, Conn.: College & University Press, 1968.
Anderson, Odis. *Health Care: Can There Be Equity?* New York: John Wiley & Son, 1972.
Angell, Marcia, "Dr. Frist to the Rescue," *American Prospect* 14 (February 1, 2003).
———. "Insufficient Credits," *American Prospect* 12 (September 2003).
Arthur, Brian. *Increasing Returns and Path Dependence in the Economy*. Ann Arbor: University of Michigan Press, 1994.
Ball, Robert. "What Medicare's Architects Had in Mind," *Health Affairs* 14 (Winter 1995): 62-73.
———. "Social Security Amendments of 1972: Summary and Legislative History," *Social Security Bulletin* 36 (March 1973): 5-11.

———. *Social Security Today and Tomorrow*. New York: Columbia University Press, 1978.

Bates, Robert, A. Grief, M. Levi, J. L. Rosenthal, and B. Weingast, eds. *Analytic Narratives*. Princeton, N.J.: Princeton University Press, 1998.

Baumgartner, Frank R., and Bryan D. Jones. *Agendas and Instability in American Politics*. Chicago: University of Chicago Press, 1993.

Behren, G. Von, N. Samuels. *The Fiscal Survey of States*. Washington, D.C.: National Association of State Budget Officers, November 2002.

Berkowitz, Edward D. *America's Welfare State from Roosevelt to Reagan*. Baltimore: Johns Hopkins University Press, 1991.

———. *Disabled Policy: America's Programs for the Handicapped*. Cambridge: Cambridge University Press, 1987.

———. "The Historical Development of Social Security in the United States." In *Social Security in the 21st Century*, ed. Eric R. Kingson and James H. Schulz. New York: Oxford University Press, 1997.

———. *Mr. Social Security: The Life of Wilbur J. Cohen*. Lawrence: University Press of Kansas, 1995.

———. *Social Security after Fifty: Successes and Failures*. New York: Greenwood Press, 1987.

Bernstein, Irving. *The Lean Years*. Boston: Houghton, Mifflin, 1960.

Biles, Brian, Geraldine Dallek, Andrew Dennington. "Medicare+Choice After Five Years: Lessons for Medicare's Future: Findings From Seven Major Cities," The Commonwealth Fund and the George Washington University Medical Center, Field Report (September 2002).

Blackstone, Erwin, and Joseph Fuhr. "Hospital Mergers and Antitrust," *Journal of Health Politics, Policy, & Law* 14 (Summer 1989): 383-403.

Blum, John. *From the Morgenthau Diaries: Years of War*. Boston: Houghton Mifflin, 1967.

Booth, Philip. *Social Security in America*. Ann Arbor: University of Michigan Press, 1973.

Bowman, Karlyn H. *Public Attitudes on Health Care Reform*. Washington, D.C.: American Enterprise Institute, 1994.

Boyd, Donald J. "The Bursting State Fiscal Bubble and State Medicaid Budgets," *Health Affairs* 22 (January/February 2003):46-61.

Brady, David and Kara Buckley. "Health Care Reform in the 103d Congress," *Journal of Health Politics, Policy & Law* 20 (Summer 1995): 447-54.

Brewer, Gary D., and Peter DeLeon. *The Foundations of Policy Analysis*. Homewood, Ill.: Dorsey Press, 1983.

Brown, J. Douglas. *An American Philosophy of Social Security*. Princeton, N.J.: Princeton University Press, 1972.

Brown, Lawrence D. *New Policies, New Politics: Government's Response to Government's Growth*. Washington, D.C.: The Brookings Institution, 1983.

———. *Politics and Health Care Organization: HMO's as Federal Policy*. Washington, D.C.: The Brookings Institution, 1983.

———. "The Politics of Medicare and Health Care Reform, Then and Now," in U.S. Department of Health and Human Services, *Health Care Financing Review* 18, "Medicare: Advancing Towards the 21st Century, 1966-1996" (Winter 1996).

———. "Technocratic Corporatism and Administrative Reform in Medicare," *Journal of Health Politics, Policy & Law* 10 (1985): 579-99.

Brown, Lawrence D., Michael Sparer. "Poor People's Progress: The Unanticipated Politics of Medicaid Policy," *Health Affairs* 22 (January/February 2003):31-44.

Bruen, B., J. Holahan. "Acceleration of Medicaid Spending Reflects Mounting Pressures." Washington: Kaiser Commission on Medicaid and the Uninsured, May 2002.

Burda, David. "What We Have Learned From DRG's," *Modern Healthcare* (October 4, 1993): 42-44.

Burrow, James G. *AMA—Voice of American Medicine.* Baltimore: Johns Hopkins University Press, 1963.

Califano, Joseph A. *Governing America.* New York: Simon & Schuster, 1981.

Cameron, David. "The Expansion of the Public Economy: A Comparative Analysis," *American Political Science Review* 72 (December 1978): 1243-61.

Campion, Frank D. *The AMA and U.S. Health Policy Since 1940.* Chicago: Chicago Review Press, 1984.

Carter, Jimmy. *Keeping Faith: Memoirs of a President.* New York: Bantam Books, 1982.

———. *Public Papers of the Presidents of the United States, 1979.* Washington, D.C.: GPO, 1980.

Carter, Richard. *The Doctor Business.* New York: Doubleday, 1958.

Cerny, Philip G. *The Changing Architecture of Politics.* London: Sage Publications, 1990.

Chase, J. Dennis. "The American Association for Labor Legislation and the Institutionalist Tradition in National Health Insurance," *Journal of Economic Issues* 28 (December 1994): 1063-90.

Christensen, S. "Medicare+Choice Provisions in the Balanced Budget Act of 1997," *Health Affairs* (July/August 1998):225-231.

Clark, Timothy B. "Congress Avoiding Political Abyss By Approving Social Security Changes," *National Journal* 15, no. 2 (March 19, 1983): 611-15.

Clinton, Hillary. *Living History.* New York: Simon & Schuster, 2003.

Coddington, Dean C., David J. Keen, and Keith D. Moore. "Cost Shifting Overshadows Employers' Cost-Containment Efforts," *Business & Health* (January 1991): 45-51.

Cohen, Wilbur J. "Federalism and Social Insurance," in *The Princeton Symposium on the America System of Social Insurance*, ed. W. Bowen. New York: McGraw-Hill, 1967.

———. "From Medicare to National Health Insurance," in *Toward a New Human Rights*, ed. David C. Warner. Austin: Lyndon B. Johnson School of Public Affairs, 1977.

Coile, R. "The Megatrends and the Backlash," *Health Care Forum Journal* (March/April 1990): 37-41.

Collier, Ruth Berins, and David Collier. *Shaping the Political Arena.* Princeton, N.J.: Princeton University Press, 1991.

Committee on the Costs of Medical Care. *Medical Care for the American People.* Chicago: University of Chicago Press, 1932.

Corning, Peter A. *The Evolution of Medicare: From Idea to Law.* Social Security Administration, Office of Research and Statistics Washington, D.C.: GPO, 1969.

Coulam, Robert F., and Gary L. Gaumer. "Medicare's Prospective Payment System: A Critical Appraisal," *Health Care Financing Review, 1991 Annual Supplement*, U.S. Department of Health and Human Services, Health Care Financing Administration (Baltimore, 1991).

Crane, M. "A New 'Malpractice Crisis'? Malpractice Rates Are Soaring Again," *Medical Economics* 9 (2001).

Dark, Taylor. "Organized Labor and the Carter Administration," in *The Presidency and Domestic Politics of Jimmy Carter*, ed. Howard Rosenbaum and A. Ugrinsky. Westport, Conn.: Greenwood Press, 1974.

Darwin, Charles. *On the Origin of the Species*. London: Cambridge University Press, 1975.

David, Paul. "Clio and the Economics of QWERTY," *American Economic Review* 75 (May 1985), 332-37.

David, Sheri I. *With Dignity: The Search for Medicare and Medicaid*. Westport, Conn.: Greenwood Press, 1985.

Davidson, Stephen, and Theodore Marmor. *The Cost of Living Longer*. Lexington, Mass.: Lexington Books, 1980.

Davis, Carolyne K. "The Federal Role in Changing Health Care Financing, Part II," *Nursing Economics* (September/October 1983): 98-104.

Davis, Karen. *National Health Insurance: Benefits, Costs, and Consequences*. Washington, D.C.: The Brookings Institution, 1975.

Davis, Karen, Cathy Schoen. "Creating Consensus on Coverage Choices," *Health Affairs* (Web Exclusive: 23 April 2003).

Demkovich, Linda. "Devising New Medicare Payment Plan May Prove Easier Than Selling It," *National Journal* 14, no. 47 (November 20, 1982): 1981-85.

———. "Who Says Congress Can't Move Fast? Just Ask the Hospitals about Medicare," *National Journal* 15, no. 14 (April 2, 1983): 704-07.

Derickson, Alan. "Health Security for All? Social Unionism and Universal Health Insurance, 1935-1958," *Journal of American History* 80 (March 1994): 1333-57.

Derthick, Martha. *Agency under Stress: The Social Security Administration in American Government*. Washington, D.C.: The Brookings Institution, 1990.

———. *Policymaking for Social Security*. Washington, D.C.: The Brookings Institution, 1979.

Dobbin, Frank R. "The Origins of Private Social Insurance: Public Policy and Fringe Benefits in America, 1920-50," *American Journal of Sociology* 97 (March 1992), 1416-50.

Dodd, Lawrence C., and Calvin Jillson, eds. *The Dynamics of America Politics*. Boulder, Colo.: Westview Press, 1994.

Edelman, Murray. *Constructing the Political Spectacle*. Chicago: University of Chicago Press, 1988.

Edwards, Jennifer, Michelle Doty, Cathy Schoen. "The Erosion of Employer-Based Health Coverage and the Threat to Workers' Health Care: Findings from the Commonwealth Fund 2002 Workplace Health Insurance Survey," Commonwealth Fund, August 2002.

Eliot, Thomas. *Recollections of the New Deal*. Boston: Northeastern University Press, 1992.

Enthoven, Alain C. "Employment-Based Health Insurance is Failing: Now What?" *Health Affairs* (Web Exclusive: 28 May 2003).

Epstein, Arnold, and David Blumenthal. "Physician Payment Reform: Past and Future," *Milibank Quarterly* 71, no. 2 (1993): 193-213.

Eubanks, Paula. "Restructuring Care," *Hospitals* 65, no. 15 (August 5, 1991): 26-28.

Evans, Peter B., Dietrich Rueschemeyer, and Theda Skocpol. *Bringing the State Back In*. Cambridge: Cambridge University Press, 1985.

Fearon, James D. "Counterfactuals and Hypothesis Testing in Political Science," *World Politics* 43 (1991): 169-95.

Feldstein, Paul J. *Health Policy Issues: An Economic Perspective on Health Reform.* Chicago: AUPHA Press, 1999.

Feder, Judith. *Medicare: The Politics of Federal Hospital Insurance.* Lexington, Mass.: Lexington Books, 1977.

———. "The Social Security Administration and Medicare: A Strategy of Implementation," in *Toward a National Health Policy: Public Policy and the Control of Health-Care Costs,* ed. Kenneth Friedman and Stuart Rakoff. Lexington, Mass.: Lexington Books, 1977.

Feder, Judith, J. Holahan, and T. Marmor, eds. *National Health Insurance: Conflicting Goals and Policy Choices.* Washington, D.C.: Urban Institute Press, 1980.

Feingold, Eugene. *Medicare: Policy and Politics.* San Francisco: Chandler Publishing Corporation, 1966.

Feldstein, Martin. *Hospital Costs and Health Insurance.* Cambridge, Mass.: Harvard University Press, 1981.

Ferejohn, John A., and James H. Kuklinski, eds. *Information and Democratic Processes.* Urbana: University of Illinois Press, 1990.

Ferrara, Peter. *Social Security: Prospects for Real Reform.* Washington, D.C.: Cato Institute, 1985.

Finbow, Robert. "Presidential Leadership or Structural Constraints? The Failure of President Carter's Health Insurance Proposals," *Presidential Studies Quarterly* 28 (Winter 1998): 169-87.

Flora, Peter, and Arnold J. Heidenheimer. *The Development of Welfare States in Europe and America.* London: Transaction Books, 1981.

Fox, Daniel. *Health Policies, Health Politics: The British and American Experience, 1911-1965.* Princeton, N.J.: Princeton University Press, 1986.

———. *Power and Illness: The Failure and Future of American Health Policy.* Berkeley: University of California Press, 1993.

Fraser, Steve, and Gary Gerstle, eds. *The Rise and Fall of the New Deal Order, 1930-1980.* Princeton, N.J.: Princeton University Press, 1989.

Friedman, Kenneth, and Stuart Rakoff, eds. *Toward a National Health Policy: Public Policy and the Control of Health-Care Costs.* Lexington, Mass.: Lexington Books, 1977.

Fuchs, Victor. *The Health Economy.* Cambridge: Cambridge University Press, 1986.

Furniss, Norman, and Timothy Tilton. *The Case for the Welfare State.* Bloomington, Ind.: Indiana University Press, 1979.

———, ed. *Futures for the Welfare State.* Indianapolis, Ind.: Indiana University Press, 1986.

Galenson, Walter, and Seymour Martin Lipset, eds. *Labor and Trade Unionism.* New York: Wiley, 1960.

Gallup. *The Gallup Public Opinion Poll, 1935-1971.* New York: Random House, 1972.

Garbarino, Joseph W. *Health Plans and Collective Bargaining.* Berkeley: University of California Press, 1960.

Glaser, William. *Health Insurance in Practice: International Variations in Financing, Benefits, and Problems.* San Francisco, Calif.: Jossey-Bass, 1991.

Gold, Marsha. "Can Managed Care and Competition Control Medicare Costs," *Health Affairs* (Web Exclusive: 2 April 2003).

Gold, Marsha, Jessica Mitler, Debra Draper, David Rousseau. "Participation of Plans and Providers in Medicaid and SCHIP Managed Care," *Health Affairs* 22 (January/ February):230-240.

Goldhagen, Daniel J. *Hitler's Willing Executioners.* New York: Knopf, 1996.

Goldmann, Franz. *Voluntary Medical Care Insurance in the United States.* New York: Columbia University Press, 1948.

Gordon, Colin. "Dead on Arrival: Health Care Reform in the United States," *Studies in Political Economy* 39 (Fall 1992): 141-59.

Gornick, Marian E., et al. "Thirty Years of Medicare: Impact on the Covered Population," in U.S. Department of Health and Human Services, *Health Care Financing Review*, "Medicare: Advancing Towards the 21st Century, 1966-1996."

Gottschalk, Marie. *The Shadow Welfare State: Labor, Business, and the Politics of Health Care in the United States.* Ithaca, N.Y.: Cornell University Press, 2000.

Gough, I. *The Political Economy of the Welfare State.* London: Macmillan, 1979.

Gourevitch, Peter. *Politics in Hard Times: Comparative Responses to International Economic Crises.* Ithaca, N.Y.: Cornell University Press, 1986.

Graebner, William. *A History of Retirement.* New Haven, Conn.: Yale University Press, 1970.

Greenberg, S.B., and Theda Skocpol. *The New Majority.* New Haven, Conn: Yale University Press, 1997.

Greve, P. "Anticipating and Controlling Rising Malpractice Insurance Costs," *Healthcare Financial Management* 56 (2002):50-56.

Gupta, Yash P. "Emerging Productivity and Cost Control in the Hospital Industry," *National Productivity Review* (Summer 1991): 351-67.

Hacker, Jacob S. "The Historical Logic of National Health Insurance," *Studies in American Political Development* 12 (Spring 1998): 57-130.

———. "National Health Care Reform: An Idea Whose Time Came and Went," *Journal of Health Politics, Policy & Law* 21 (Winter 1996): 647-96.

———. *The Road to Nowhere: The Genesis of President Clinton's Plan for Health Security.* Princeton, N.J.: Princeton University Press, 1997.

Hacker, Jacob, and Theda Skocpol. "The New Politics of U.S. Health Policy," *Journal of Health Politics, Policy & Law* 22 (April 1997): 315-38.

Hall, Peter. *The Political Power of Economic Ideas: Keynesianism Across Nations.* Princeton, N.J.: Princeton University Press, 1989.

———, and Rosemary C.R. Taylor, "Political Science and the Three Institutionalisms," *Political Studies* 44 (1996): 936-57.

Halpern, Martin. "Jimmy Carter and the UAW: Failure of an Alliance," *Presidential Studies Quarterly* 26 (Summer 1996): 755-77.

Harris, Richard. *A Sacred Trust.* New York: New American Library, 1966.

Harrop, Martin. *Power and Policy in Liberal Democracies.* Cambridge: Cambridge University Press, 1992.

Hartz, Louis. *The Liberal Tradition in America.* New York: Harcourt, Brace, 1955.

Hayes, M. *Incrementalism and Public Policy.* New York: Longman, 1992.

Heclo, Hugh. "The Clinton Health Plan: Historical Perspective," *Health Affairs* 14 (Spring 1995): 86-98.

———. *Modern Social Politics in Britain and Sweden.* New Haven, Conn.: Yale University Press, 1974.

Heffler, Stephen, Sheila Smith, Sean Keehan, M. Kent Clemens, Greg Won, Mark Zezza. "Health Spending Projections for 2002-2012," *Health Affairs* (Web Exclusive: 7 February 2003).

Heidenheimer, Arnold, H. Heclo, and Carolyn T. Adams. *Comparative Public Policy: The Politics of Social Choice in Europe and America.* New York: St. Martin's Press, 1983.

Heidenheimer, Arnold, and Peter Flora. *The Development of Welfare States in Europe and America.* London: Transaction Books, 1981.

Heirich, Max. *Rethinking Health Care.* Boulder, Colo.: Westview Press, 1998.

———, and Marilynn M. Rosenthall. *Health Policy.* Boulder, Colo.: Westview Press, 1998.

Heller, W. *New Dimensions of Political Economy.* Cambridge, Mass.: Harvard University Press, 1966.

Hill, Ian, Amy Westpfahl Lutzky. "Is There a Hole in the Bucket? Understanding SCHIP Retention," Assessing the New Federalism, Occasional Paper No. 67 (Urban Institute: May 2003).

Himmelfarb, Richard. *Catastrophic Politics: The Rise and Fall of the Medicare Catastrophic Coverage Act of 1988.* University Park: Pennsylvania State University Press, 1995.

Hirshfield, Daniel S. *The Lost Reform: The Campaign for Compulsory Health Insurance in the United States from 1932 to 1943.* Cambridge, Mass.: Harvard University Press, 1970.

Holtzman, Abraham. *The Townsend Movement: A Political Study.* New York: Bookman Associates, 1963.

Howard, Christopher. *The Hidden Welfare State: Tax Expenditures and Social Policy in the United States.* Princeton, N.J.: Princeton University Press, 1997.

Howell, Embry, Ruth Almeida, Lisa Dubay, Genevieve Kenney. "Early Experience with Covering Uninsured Parents Under SCHIP," Series A, No. A-51, Urban Institute (Washington, D.C.: May 2002).

Huntington, Samuel. "The Clash of Civilizations?" *Foreign Affairs* 72 (Summer 1993): 22-50.

Iglehart, John K. "The Dilemma of Medicaid," *New England Journal of Medicine* 348 (May 22, 2003):2140-2148.

Ikenberry, John. "History's Heavy Hand: Institutions and Politics of the State." Paper presented at the Conference on "New Institutionalism," University of Maryland, October 14-15, 1994.

Immergut, Ellen M. *Health Politics: Interests and Institutions in Western Europe.* Cambridge: Cambridge University Press, 1992.

Jacobs, David. "The UAW and the Committee for National Health Insurance," in *Advances in Industrial and Labor Relations* 4. Greenwich: JAI Press, 1987.

Jacobs, Lawrence R. *The Health of Nations: Public Opinion and the Making of Health Policy in Britain and the United States.* Ithaca, N.Y.: Cornell University Press, 1993.

Jacoby, Melissa, Teresa Sullivan, Elizabeth Warren. "Rethinking the Debates Over Health Care Financing: Evidence from the Bankruptcy Courts," *New York University Law Review* 76 (May 2001):375-412.

James, Tom, and David B. Nash. "Health Maintenance Organizations: A New Development or the Emperor's Old Clothes?" in *Readings in American Health Care*, ed. William G. Rothstein. Madison, Wis.: University of Wisconsin Press, 1995.

Javits, Jacob. *The Autobiography of a Public Man.* Boston: Houghton Mifflin, 1981.

Johnson, Haynes, and David S. Broder. *The System: The American Way of Politics at the Breaking Point.* New York: Little, Brown & Company, 1996.

Judis, John B. "Abandoned Surgery: Business and the Failure of Health Care Reform," *American Prospect* 21 (Spring 1995): 65-73.

Kahn, Chip, Hanns Kuttner. "Budget Bills and Medicare Policy: The Politics of the BBA," *Health Affairs* 18 (January/February 1999):37-47.

Karger, H., and David Stoesz. *American Social Welfare Policy.* New York: Longman, 1998.

King, Gary, Robert Keohane, and Sidney Verba. *Designing Social Inquiry: Scientific Inference in Qualitative Research.* Princeton: Princeton University Press, 1994.

Kingdon, John. *Agendas, Alternatives, and Public Policies.* Boston: Little, Brown & Company, 1984.

Kooijman, Jaap. . . . *And the Pursuit of National Health: The Incremental Strategy toward National Health Insurance in the United States.* Amsterdam: Rodopi, 1999.

———. "Soon or Later On: Franklin D. Roosevelt and National Health Insurance, 1933-1945," *Presidential Studies Quarterly* 29 (June 1999): 336-54.

Krasner, Stephen. *Defending the National Interest.* Princeton, N.J.: Princeton University Press, 1978.

———. "Sovereignty: An Institutional Perspective," *Comparative Political Studies* 21 (April 1988): 66-94.

Kronick, T. Gilmer. "Explaining the Decline in Health Insurance Coverage, 1979-1995," *Health Affairs* (March/April 1999):30-47.

Ku, Leighton. "The Number of Americans Without Health Insurance Rose in 2001 and Appears to be Continuing to Rise in 2002," Center on Budget and Policy Priorities (Washington, D.C.: October 8, 2002).

Laham, Nicholas. *Why the United States Lacks a National Health Insurance Program.* London: Praeger, 1993.

Laslett, John, and Seymour Martin Lipset. *Failure of a Dream? Essays in the History of American Socialism.* Los Angeles: University of California Press, 1984.

Lave, Judith R., and Lester B. Lave. *The Hospital Construction Act: An Evaluation of the Hill-Burton Program, 1948-1973.* Washington, D.C.: American Enterprise Institute, 1974.

Levi, Margaret. "Producing an Analytic Narrative," in *Critical Comparisons in Politics and Culture,* ed. John Bowen and Roger Peterson. New York: Cambridge University Press, 1999.

Light, Paul. *Artful Work: The Politics of Social Security Reform.* New York: Random House, 1985.

Lindblom, Charles. *Politics and Markets: The World's Political-Economic Systems.* New York: Basic Books, 1977.

Lipset, Seymour Martin. *American Exceptionalism: A Double-Edged Sword.* New York: W. W. Norton & Company, 1996.

Lowi, Theodore J. "American Business, Public Policy Case-Studies, and Political Theory," *World Politics* (1964): 677-715.

———, and A. Stone. *Nationalizing Government: Public Policies in America.* London: Sage Publications, 1978.

Lubove, Roy. *The Struggle for Social Security, 1900-1935.* Cambridge, Mass.: Harvard University Press, 1968.

MacColl, William. *Group Practice and Prepayment of Medical Care.* Washington, D.C.: Public Affairs Press, 1966.

Mann, Thomas, and Norman Ornstein, eds. *Intensive Care: How Congress Shapes Health Policy.* Washington, D.C.: The Brookings Institution, 1995.

March, James G., and Johan P. Olsen. "The New Institutionalism: Organizational Factors in Political Life," *American Political Science Review* 78 (September 1984): 734-49.

Marmor, Theodore R. *The Politics of Medicare.* Chicago: Aldine Publishing Company, 1970.

———. *The Politics of Medicare,* 2d ed. New York: Aldine de Gruyter, 2000.

————. *Understanding Health Care Reform.* New Haven, Conn.: Yale University Press, 1994.

Marmor, Theodore R., and Jerry Mashaw, eds. *Social Security: Beyond the Rhetoric of Crisis.* Princeton, N.J.: Princeton University Press, 1988.

Mashaw, Jerry L. *The Bureaucratic State.* New Haven, Conn.: Yale University Press, 1983.

Matusow, Allen J. *Nixon's Economy: Booms, Busts, Dollars, and Votes.* Lawrence: University Press of Kansas, 1998.

Mayhew, David. *The Electoral Connection.* New Haven, Conn.: Yale University Press, 1974.

McClure, Arthur F. *The Truman Administration and the Problems of Postwar Labor, 1945-58.* Rutherford, N.J.: Fairleigh Dickinson Press, 1969.

Mello, Michelle, David Studdert, Troyen Brennan. "The New Medical Malpractice Crisis." *New England Journal of Medicine* 348 (June 5, 2003):2281-2284.

Miller, Joel E. "Déjà Vu All Over Again: The Soaring Cost of Private Health Insurance and Its Impact on Consumers and Employers." *National Coalition On Health Care.* Washington, D.C.: May 2000.

Mitchell, W. L. "Social Security Legislation in the 86th Congress," *Social Security Bulletin* (November 1960).

Mongan, James. "Anatomy and Physiology of Health Care Reform's Failure," *Health Affairs* 14 (Spring 1995): 99-101.

Moon, Marilyn. *Medicare Now and in the Future.* Washington, D.C.: Urban Institute Press, 1996.

Moore, Barrington. *Social Origins of Dictatorship and Democracy.* Harmondsworth: Penguin, 1973.

Moore, Perry. *Evaluating Health Maintenance Organizations.* New York: Quorum Books, 1991.

Morone, James. "The Administration of Health Care Reform." *Journal of Health Politics, Policy & Law* 19 (1994): 233-37.

————. "Nativism, Hollow Corporations, and Managed Competition," *Journal of Health Politics, Policy & Law* 20 (Summer 1995): 391-98.

Morone, James, and Gary Belkin, eds. *The Politics of Health Care Reform.* Durham, N.C.: Duke University Press, 1994.

Mortimer, Rick, "What's Happening to the Cost and Quality of Medical Malpractice Insurance," *Cost and Quality Journal* (March 1998).

Mucciaroni, Gary. *Reversals of Fortune: Public Policy and Private Interests.* Washington, D.C.: The Brookings Institution, 1995.

Munts, Raymond. *Bargaining for Health: Labor Unions, Health Insurance, and Medical Care.* Madison, Wis.: University of Wisconsin Press, 1960.

Myers, Robert J. *Medicare.* Bryn Mawr, Pa.: McCahan Foundation, 1970.

————. *Social Security.* Bryn Mawr, Pa.: McCahan Foundation, 1975.

————. *Social Insurance and Allied Government.* Homewood, Ill.: R. D. Irwin, 1965.

Nash, Gerald, Noel H. Pugach, and Richard F. Tomasson. *Social Security, the First Half-Century.* Albuquerque: University of New Mexico Press, 1988.

"National Health Insurance: A Concept Whose Time Has Come," *Journal of Accountancy* 138 (July 1974), 25.

Navarro, Vicente. "Why Congress Did Not Enact Health Care Reform," *Journal of Health Politics, Policy & Law* 20 (Summer 1995): 455-62.

————. *Why the United States Does Not Have a National Health Program.* Amityville, N.Y.: Baywood Pub. Co., 1992.

Newhouse, Joseph P., Charles E. Phelps, and Williams B. Schwartz. *Policy Options and the Impact of National Health Insurance.* Santa Monica, Calif.: Rand, June 1974.

Nixon, Richard. *Public Papers of the Presidents of the United States.* Washington, D.C.: U.S. GPO, 1975.

————. *Six Crises.* Garden City, N.Y.: Doubleday, 1962.

North, Douglass C. *Institutions, Institutional Change, and Economic Performance.* New York: Cambridge University Press, 1990.

Numbers, Ronald L. *Almost Persuaded: American Physicians and Compulsory Health Insurance, 1912-1920.* Baltimore, Md.: Johns Hopkins University Press, 1978.

Oberlander, Jonathan. *Medicare and the American State.* Ph.D. dissertation, Yale University. Available from UMI Dissertation Service, Ann Arbor, 1995.

————. "One Dimensional," *American Prospect* (Web Feature: February 2003).

————. *The Political Life of Medicare.* Chicago: The University of Chicago Press, 2003.

Oliver, Tom. *Conceptualizing the Challenges of Public Sector Entrepreneurship.* Westport, Conn.: Praeger, 1996.

Olson, Mancur, ed. *A New Approach to the Economics of Health Care.* Washington, D.C.: American Enterprise Institute, 1980.

Pauly, Mark V., ed. *National Health Insurance: What Now, What Later, What Never?* Washington, D.C.: AEI Press, 1980.

Pechman, J., Henry J. Aaron, and M. K. Taussig. *Social Security: Perspectives for Reform.* Washington, D.C.: The Brookings Institution, 1968.

Perkins, Frances. *The Roosevelt I Knew.* New York: The Viking Press, 1946.

Peterson, Mark A. "Congress in the 1990s: From Iron Triangles to Policy Networks," in *The Politics of Health Care Reform,* ed. James A. Morone and Gary S. Belkin. Durham, N.C.: Duke University Press, 1994.

————. "Institutional Change and the Health Politics of the 1990s," *American Behavioral Scientist* 36 (July-August 1993): 782-802.

————. "The Politics of Health Care Policy: Overreaching in an Age of Polarization," in *The Social Divide: Political Parties and the Future of Activist Government,* ed. Margaret Weir. Washington, D.C.: The Brookings Institution, 1998.

Pierson, Paul. *Dismantling the Welfare State? Reagan, Thatcher, and the Politics of Retrenchment.* Cambridge: Cambridge University Press, 1994.

————. "Increasing Returns, Path Dependence, and the Study of Politics." Program for the Study of Germany and Europe, Working Paper Series 7.7, Center for European Studies, Harvard University, September 1, 1997.

————. "Increasing Returns, Path Dependence, and the Study of Politics," *American Political Science Review* 94 (June 2000): 251-67.

————. "Not Just What, But When: Timing and Sequence in Political Processes," *Studies in American Political Development* 14 (Spring 2000): 79-92.

————. "When Effect Becomes Cause: Policy Feedback and Political Change," *World Politics* 45 (July 1993): 595-628.

Piore, Michael, and Charles Sabel. *The Second Industrial Divide.* New York: Basic Books, 1984.

Poen, Monte M. *Harry S. Truman versus the Medical Lobby.* Columbia: University of Missouri Press, 1979.

Przeworski, Adam. *Capitalism and Social Democracy.* Cambridge: Cambridge University Press, 1985.

Przeworski, Adam, and M. Wallerstein. "The Structure of Class Conflict in Democratic Capitalist Societies," *American Political Science Review* 76 (1982): 215-38.

Putnam, Robert. *Making Democracy Work.* Princeton, N.J.: Princeton University Press, 1993.

Quadagno, Jill. "Generational Equity and the Politics of the Welfare State," *Politics and Society* 17 (1997): 353-76.

———. "Theories of the Welfare State," *Annual Review of Sociology* 13 (1987): 109-28.

Rakich, Jonathon S., and Edmund R. Becker. "United States Physician Payment Reform" *Health Care Management Review* 17, no. 1 (Winter 1992): 9-19

Rapport, John, Robert Robertson, and Bruce Stuart. *Understanding Health Economics.* Rockville, Md.: Aspen Systems Corporation, 1982.

Rauch, Jonathon. *Demosclerosis: The Silent Killer of American Government.* New York: Times Books, 1994.

Reagan, Michael D. *The Accidental System: Health Care Policy in America.* Boulder, Colo.: Westview Press, 1999.

———. *Curing the Crisis: Options for American's Health Care.* Boulder, Colo.: Westview Press, 1992.

Reardon, Jack, and Laurie Reardon. "The Restructuring of the Hospital Services Industry," *Journal of Economic Issues* 29 (December 1995): 1064-81.

Reichard, Gary W. *The Reaffirmation of Republicanism: Eisenhower and the Eighty-Third Congress.* Knoxville: University of Tennessee Press, 1975.

Reschovsky, James, Peter Cunningham. "CHIPing Away at the Problem of Uninsured Children," *Issue Brief 14* (Washington, D.C.: Center for Studying Health System Change, August 1998).

Rimlinger, Gaston. *Welfare Policy and Industrialization in Europe and America.* New York: Wiley, 1971.

Robinson, James C. "The End of Managed Care," *JAMA, The Journal of the American Medical Association* 285 (May 23/30, 2001):2622-2628.

Romer, Paul M. "Increasing Returns and Long-Run Growth," *Journal of Political Economy* 94 (1986): 1002-37.

Rose, Richard, and Phillip L. Davies. *Inheritance in Public Policy.* New Haven, Conn.: Yale University Press, 1994.

Rose, Richard, and B. Guy Peters. *The Juggernaut of Incrementalism: A Comparative Perspective on the Growth of Public Policy.* Glasgow: University of Strathclyde, 1978.

Rosenbaum, H., and A. Ugrinsky, eds. *The Presidency and Domestic Politics of Jimmy Carter.* Westport, Conn.: Greenwood Press, 1974.

Rosenbaum, S. "Medicaid," *New England Journal of Medicine* 346 (2002):635-640.

Rosenthal, M., and M. Frenkel. *Health Care Systems.* Boulder, Colo.: Westview Press, 1992.

Rothman, David. "A Century of Failure: Health Care Reform in America," *Journal of Health Politics, Policy & Law* (Summer 1993): 271-86.

Rowland, Diane, James Tallon Jr. "Medicaid: Lessons From a Decade," *Health Affairs* 22 (January/February 2003):138-144.

Rueschemeyer, Dietrich, Evelyne Huber Stephens, and Johns D. Stephens. *Critical Comparisons in Politics and Culture.* Chicago: University of Chicago Press, 1992.

Rueschemeyer, Dietrich, and Theda Skocpol. *States, Social Knowledge, and the Origins of Modern Social Policies.* Princeton, N.J.: Princeton University Press, 1996.

Ruggie, Mary. *Realignments in the Welfare State: Health Policy in the United States, Britain & Canada.* New York: Columbia University Press, 1997.

Rushefsky, Mark, and Kant Patel. *Politics, Power and Policy Making: The Case of Health Care Reform in the 1990s.* Armonk, N.Y.: M. E. Sharpe, 1998.

Russell, Louise B. *Medicare's New Hospital Payment System: Is It Working?* Washington, D.C.: The Brookings Institution, 1989.

Ryan, Jennifer M. "SCHIP Turns Five: Taking Stock, Moving Ahead," National Health Policy Forum, Issue Brief No. 781, George Washington University: August 15, 2002.

Samuelson, Paul. "On Social Security," *Newsweek*, February 13, 1967, 88.

Schattschneider, E. E. *Politics, Pressures and the Tariff.* New York: Prentice-Hall, 1935.

———. *The Semi-Sovereign People: A Realist's View of Democracy in America.* New York: Harcourt Brace Jovanovich, 1975.

Schick, Allen. "How a Bill Did not Become a Law," in *Intensive Care: How Congress Shapes Health Policy,* ed. Thomas Mann and Norman Ornstein. Washington, D.C.: The Brookings Institution, 1995.

Schlesinger, Arthur M., Jr. *A Thousand Days: John F. Kennedy in the White House.* Boston: Houghton Mifflin, 1965.

Schumpeter, Joseph. *Capitalism, Socialism, and Democracy.* New York: Harper & Row, 2nd ed., 1947.

Scott, Richard. *Institutions and Organizations.* Thousand Oaks, Calif.: Sage, 1995.

Scott, Richard, Martin Ruef, Peter Mendel, and Carol Caronna. *Institutional Change and Healthcare Organizations: From Professional to Managed Care.* Chicago: University of Chicago Press, 2000.

Shafer, Byron E., ed. *Is America Different? A New Look at American Exceptionalism.* Oxford: Clarendon Press, 1991.

Shortell, Stephen, Ellen Morrison, and Bernard Friedman. *Strategic Choices for America's Hospitals.* San Francisco, Calif.: Jossey-Bass, 1990.

Skidmore, Max. *Medicare and the American Rhetoric of Reconciliation.* Tuscaloosa: University of Alabama Press, 1970.

Skocpol, Theda. *Boomerang: Health Care Reform and the Turn Against Government.* New York: W. W. Norton & Co., 1996.

———. "Is the Time Finally Ripe? Health Insurance Reforms in the 1990s," *Journal of Health Politics, Policy & Law* 18 (Fall 1993): 531-50.

———. *Protecting Soldiers and Mothers: The Political Origins of Social Policy in the United States.* Cambridge, Mass.: Harvard University Press, 1992.

———. *Social Policy in the United States.* Princeton, N.J.: Princeton University Press, 1995.

Skowronek, Stephen. *Building a New American State: The Expansion of National Administrative Capacities, 1877-1920.* Cambridge: Cambridge University Press, 1982.

Smith, David G. *Paying for Medicare: The Politics of Reform.* New York: Aldine de Gruyter, 1992.

Social Security Board. *Social Security in America.* Washington, D.C.: GPO, 1937.

Somers, Anne R., and Herman M. Somers. *Doctors, Patients, and Health Insurance.* Washington, D.C.: The Brookings Institution, 1961.

———. *Health and Health Care: Policies in Perspective.* Germantown, Md.: Aspen Systems Corporation, 1977.

———. *Medicare and the Hospitals.* Washington, D.C.: The Brookings Institution, 1967.

Spiegel, Allen D., and Simon Podair. *Medicaid: Lessons for National Health Insurance.* Rockville, Md.: Aspen Systems Corporation, 1975.

Starr, Paul. *The Social Transformation of American Medicine.* New York: Basic Books, 1984.

———. "What Happened to Health Care Reform?" *American Prospect* 20 (Winter 1995): 20-31.

Steinmo, Sven, "American Exceptionalism Reconsidered," in *The Dynamics of America Politics*, ed. L. C. Dodd and C. Jillson. Boulder, Colo.: Westview Press, 1994.

Steinmo, Sven, and Jon Watts. "It's the Institutions, Stupid! Why Comprehensive National Health Insurance Always Fails in American," *Journal of Health Politics, Policy & Law* 20 (Summer 1995): 329-72.

Steinmo, Sven, Kathleen Thelen, and Frank Longstreth. *Structuring Politics*. Cambridge: Cambridge University Press, 1992.

Stephens, John. *The Transformation from Capitalism to Socialism*. London: Macmillan, 1979.

Stevens, Beth. "Blurring the Boundaries: How the Federal Government Has Influenced Welfare Benefits in the Private Sector," in *The Politics of Social Policy in the United States*, ed. M. Weir, A. Orloff, and T. Skocpol. Princeton, N.J.: Princeton University Press, 1988.

Stevens, Rosemary. *American Medicine and the Public Interest*. New Haven, Conn.: Yale University Press, 1971.

———. *In Sickness and in Wealth: American Hospitals in the Twentieth Century*. New York: Basic Books, 1989.

Stone, Deborah. *The Disabled State*. Philadelphia: Temple University Press, 1984.

Strahan, Randall. *New Ways and Means: Reform and Change in a Congressional Committee*. Chapel Hill, N.C.: University of North Carolina Press, 1990.

Strunk, Bradley, Paul Ginsburg, Jon Gabel. "Tracking Health Care Costs: Growth Accelerates Again in 2001," *Health Affairs* (Web Exclusive: 25 September 2002).

Sundquist, James. *Politics and Policy: The Eisenhower, Kennedy, and Johnson Years*. Washington, D.C.: The Brookings Institution, 1968.

Svahn, John, and Mary Ross. "Social Security Amendments of 1983: Legislative History and Summary of Provisions," *Social Security Bulletin* 46, no. 7 (July 1983): 3-48.

Tetlock, Philip E., and Aaron Belkin. *Counterfactual Thought Experiments in World Politics*. Princeton, N.J.: Princeton University Press, 1996.

Thelen, Kathleen. "Historical Institutionalism in Comparative Politics," paper presented at the 1998 American Political Science Association Annual Meeting, Boston.

———. "Historical Institutionalism in Comparative Politics," *Annual Review of Political Science* 2 (1999): 369-404.

———. "Timing and Temporality in the Analysis of Institutional Evolution and Change," *Studies in American Political Development* 14 (Spring 2000): 101-08.

Truman, Harry S. *Public Papers of the President of the United States, 1949*. Washington, D.C.: GPO, 1950.

———. *Years of Trial and Hope, 1946-1953*. New York: Doubleday, 1956.

Tufte, Edward. *Political Control of the Economy*. Princeton, N.J.: Princeton University Press, 1978.

Tuohy, C. *Accidental Logics*. New York: Oxford University Press, 1999.

Van Gorkom, J. W. *Social Security Revisited*. Washington, D.C.: American Enterprise Institute, 1977.

Wainess, Flint J. "The Ways and Means of National Health Care Reform, 1974 and Beyond," *Journal of Health Politics, Policy & Law* 24 (April 1999): 305-33.

Waldman, Saul. *National Health Insurance Proposals: Provisions of Bills Introduced in the 93rd Congress as of October 1973*. Washington, D.C.: Department of HEW, Social Security Administration, Office of Research and Statistics.

Warner, David C. *Toward New Human Rights*. University of Texas at Austin, Lyndon B. Johnson School of Public Affairs, 1977.

Warren, Elizabeth, Teresa Sullivan, Melissa Jacoby. "Medical Problems and Bankruptcy Problems," Harvard Law School, Public Law Working Paper 8 (April 2000).

Weaver, R. Kent. *Automatic Government: The Politics of Indexation.* Washington, D.C.: The Brookings Institution, 1988.

Weaver, R. Kent, and Bert A. Rockman. *Do Institutions Matter? Government Capabilities in the United States and Abroad.* Washington, D.C.: The Brookings Institution, 1993.

Weber, Max. *On Charisma and Institution Building.* Chicago: University of Chicago Press, 1968.

Weil, Alan. "There's Something About Medicaid," *Health Affairs* 22 (January/February 2003):13-30.

Weir, Margaret. *Politics and Jobs: The Boundaries of Employment Policy in the United States.* Princeton, N.J.: Princeton University Press, 1992.

———, ed. *The Social Divide: Political Parties and the Future of Activist Government* Washington, D.C.: The Brookings Institution, 1998.

Weir, Margaret, Shola Orloff, and Theda Skocpol. *The Politics of Social Policy in the United States.* Princeton, N.J.: Princeton University Press, 1988.

Weissert, C. S., and W. G. Weissert. *Governing Health: The Politics of Health Policy.* Baltimore, Md.: Johns Hopkins University Press, 1996.

White, Joseph. *Competing Solutions: American Health Care Proposals and International Experience.* Washington, D.C.: The Brookings Institution, 1995.

———. "The Horses and the Jumps: Comments on the Health Care Reform Steeplechase," *Journal of Health Politics, Policy & Law* 20 (Summer 1995): 373-84.

Wickizer, Thomas, and Paul Feldstein. "The Impact of HMO Competition on Private Health Insurance Premiums, 1985-92," *Inquiry* 32 (Fall 1995): 241-51.

Wildavsky, Aaron. *The Politics of the Budgetary Process.* Boston: Little Brown, 1984.

Wilensky, Gail R. "Interview: Thinking Outside the Box: A Conversation with John Breaux," *Health Affairs* (Web Exclusive: 5 March 2003).

Williams, T. Harry. *Huey Long.* New York: Vintage Books, 1969.

Witte, Edwin. *The Development of the Social Security Act.* Madison: University of Wisconsin Press, 1962.

———. "Excerpts from Address at the Meeting of the Catholic Economic Association at Chicago, December 28, 1958," *Review of Social Economy* 17 (March 1959): 31-32.

Wolinsky, H., and Tom Brune. *The Serpent on the Staff.* New York: G. P. Putnam's Sons, 1994.

Wolkstein, Irwin. "Medicare's Financial Status—How Did We Get There?" in *Conference on the Future of Medicare*, Committee on Ways and Means, U.S. House of Representatives, 98th Congress, 1st Session (November 29, 1983).

Zelizer, Julian E. *Taxing America: Wilbur D. Mills, Congress, and the State, 1945-1975.* Cambridge: Cambridge University Press, 1998.

Zelman, Walter, and Lawrence D. Brown. "Interview: Looking Back on Health Care Reform: 'No Easy Choices'," *Health Affairs* 17 (November/December 1998):61-68.

Zuckerman, Stephen. "Medical Malpractice: Claims, Legal Costs, and the Practice of Defensive Medicine," *Health Affairs* 3 (1988):128-134.

Zysman, John. "How Institutions Create Historically Rooted Trajectories of Growth," *Journal of Industrial and Corporate Change* 3 (November 1994):243-83.

INDEX

Abernethy, David, 170, 172, 173
Achenbaum, Andrew, 4
Aetna lawsuit, 151
AFL–CIO, 65, 66, 81, 90, 92, 93
Albert, Carl, 97
Altman, Drew E., 148
Altmeyer, Arthur, 24, 33-34, 37, 42, 81
American Association of Retired
  Persons (AARP), 127, 177
American exceptionalism, 2
American Hospital Association (AHA),
  68, 117, 119
American Medical Association (AMA),
  xi, 7, 10, 19-20, 21, 22, 24, 25, 31,
  33-34, 36, 37-38, 41, 46, 47, 54, 61,
  66, 68, 93, 94, 140; declining
  political influence, 64-65, 82;
  Eldercare proposal, 68-69; first
  defeat over disability insurance, 55-
  56; Medicredit proposal, 82, 88, 92,
  93, 94, 95, 96; opposition to
  Medicare, 64-66, 68-69, 112
Angell, Marcia, 173

Balanced Budget Act (1997), 162,
Ball, Robert, 32, 70, 81, 93, 112-113
Bamberger, Lee, 65, 66
Bentsen, Lloyd, 169
Berkowitz, Edward, xii, 53-54, 99, 155
Berra, Yogi, 149
Better-care, 69
Beveridge Plan, 35, 43n28
Biemiller, Andy, 92-93
Blue Cross/Blue Shield, xii, 8, 9, 39,
  49, 56, 66, 68, 73, 74
Boorstin, Bob, 168
Borah, William, 24

Bradley, Wayne, 93
Brady, David, 129
Breaux, John, 147, 174
Brindle, James, 46, 65
Bromberg, Michael, 115-116
Brown, Lawrence, 62, 121
Buckley, Karen, 129
Budget deficits, 116-117, 122
Burke, Sheila, 171
Burleson, Omar, 91, 92
Bush, Sr., George, 177
Bush, Jr., George, 147, 173
Business Roundtable, 130, 168

Califano, Joseph, 98
Carstenson, Blue, 66-67
Carter, Jimmy, 1, 97, 98, 99
Champion, Hale, 98-99
Chamber of Commerce, 52, 130, 151
Clinton, Bill, xi, xii, 1, 2 4, 10, 109,
  110, 122-125, 126, 127, 128, 129,
  130, 141, 142, 143, 167-172.
  See also Health Security Act
Clinton, Hillary, 167-172
Cohen, Wilbur, 24, 33, 36, 62, 74n1,
  81, 83, 84
Collective bargaining, 8, 45-47, 53, 56,
  65, 82, 140, 141
Committee on Economic Security
  (CES), 17, 18-19, 20, 21, 23, 24,
  25, 26n18, 33; members of, 26n8
Committee on Medical Care, 33
Congressional Budget Office (CBO),
  122, 129
Conyers, John, 173
Corman, James, 94
Cost-shifting, 9, 112, 118-121, 129

ABOUT THE AUTHOR

Rick Mayes is an assistant professor of public policy in the University of Richmond's department of political science. He is also a faculty research fellow at the Nicholas C. Petris Center on Healthcare Markets and Consumer Welfare at the University of California, Berkeley. Previously he was a lecturer and National Institute of Mental Health postdoctoral trainee at the University of California, Berkeley School of Public Health from 2000 to 2002. His professional experience has included work on Medicaid policy for President George Bush in the White House Office of Intergovernmental Affairs in 1992, as well as being an aide in the Federal Affairs Division (Health Care Team) of the American Association of Retired Persons during the Clinton reform effort in 1994. His writings have appeared in *Health Affairs*, the *Journal of Policy History*, *Applied Health Economics & Health Policy*, and the *Journal of Health Care Law & Policy*. He received his Ph.D. from the University of Virginia, and his B.A. from the University of Richmond. He and his family live in Richmond, Virginia.